# Complement

# Complement
## Clinical Aspects and Relevance to Disease

**B. PAUL MORGAN**
*Department of Medical Biochemistry,
University of Wales College of Medicine,
Cardiff, UK*

ACADEMIC PRESS
Harcourt Brace Jovanovich, Publishers
London  San Diego  New York
Boston  Sydney  Tokyo  Toronto

*This book is printed on acid-free paper*

ACADEMIC PRESS LIMITED
24–28 Oval Road
London NW1 7DX

*United States Edition published by*
ACADEMIC PRESS INC.
San Diego, CA 92101

Copyright © 1990 by
ACADEMIC PRESS LIMITED

*All Rights Reserved*
No part of this book may be reproduced in any form
by photostat, microfilm, or by any other means,
without written permission from the publishers

**British Library Cataloguing in Publication Data**
Is available

ISBN 0–12–506955–3

Typeset by Columns Design and
Production Services Ltd, Reading
Printed in Great Britain by
TJ Press (Padstow) Ltd, Padstow, Cornwall

# Contents

| | |
|---|---|
| Foreword | vii |
| Acknowledgements | ix |

CHAPTER ONE
The Complement System   1

CHAPTER TWO
The Biological Effects of Complement Activation   36

CHAPTER THREE
The Genetics of Complement   57

CHAPTER FOUR
Complement Deficiencies and Disease   78

CHAPTER FIVE
Complement and Infectious Diseases   97

CHAPTER SIX
Complement and Renal Disease   112

CHAPTER SEVEN
Complement and Rheumatic Disease   130

CHAPTER EIGHT
Complement in Neurological and Muscular
   Diseases  141

CHAPTER NINE
Complement and Dermatological Diseases  156

CHAPTER TEN
Complement in Iatrogenic and Post-traumatic
   Syndromes  169

CHAPTER ELEVEN
Complement in Other Diseases  179

CHAPTER TWELVE
Complement Measurement and Potential for
   Therapeutic Manipulation  193

Index  209

# Foreword

Like all the components of the immune system, complement first appeared in early vertebrate evolution and became a subject of scientific study at the end of the nineteenth century. Recognised originally as an activity of the plasma needed for the lysis of red cells and the killing of bacteria it rapidly became clear that complement was a highly complex interacting system of multiple components. In the 1940s and 50s it fell victim to an attempt to define the system in terms of kinetic analysis and acquired the reputation of an arcane mystery which gave rise to the unloved status to which Paul Morgan refers in his first sentence!

This has now been unfair for a long time. In the 1960s the components of the complement system were first isolated as proteins and as antigens and the major pathways of complement activation began to be worked out. In the 1980s the full force of molecular biology was applied to the subject and virtually all the components and related proteins have now been cloned and sequenced. The biochemistry, the genetics and the functions of the system are now reasonably well understood although much remains to be clarified. While complement indeed turns out to be very complex — and very elegant — it is no more so than the major histocompatibility complex or the cytokines or, indeed, the membrane markers on lymphocytes. For all those who have come to terms with these aspects of the immune system, complement should hold no particular terrors.

To prove this point Dr Paul Morgan's excellent book is both welcome and timely. It deals with the subject in a logical and clear way going from its history to its biochemistry, to its functions and genetics and to its medical implications. The main emphasis is on the functional and medical aspects and it should provide an excellent text not only for those who are conversant with the field and would like a readable and non-turgid account of the subject but also to the larger number who know that complement is involved in a number of diseases and that the complement levels are sometimes useful to measure but who would really like to know what it is that is measured and why.

Paul Morgan's enthusiasm for the subject shines through the writing and illuminates the reading. Whether or not he succeeds in making complement more loved, I am sure he will make it less misunderstood.

Professor P. J. Lachmann

# Acknowledgements

I am indebted to the members of my research group for criticising parts of the text and for keeping the laboratory running while my attention was elsewhere. I thank the many colleagues who have encouraged me to write this text and allowed me to use their illustrations and the Editorial staff at Academic Press for their help and patience. The original figures were made comprehensible by Adrian Shaw and Janice Sharp.

Without the unfailing support of Celia, Lewys, Lloyd and Rhys this book would never have been contemplated. I dedicate this book, my first but hopefully not my last, to them and to my parents, Barbara and Donald, who have always provided gentle guidance and confidence.

CHAPTER ONE

# The Complement System

## 1.1 INTRODUCTION

The complement system, through no fault of its own, is unloved. The majority of doctors and scientists who encounter the system during their training are horrified by the bizarre terminology and confused by the complex entangling and entwining of pathways which typify most attempts to represent the system schematically. The result of this unfortunate state of affairs is that few scientists and even fewer clinicians clear this first hurdle and discover more about the absorbing biochemical intricacies and clinical importance of the complement system. The aim of this book is to give these busy individuals a helping hand by providing a complete and concise account of the complement system and its importance in disease.

In order to explain how our current knowledge has evolved and to clarify historical incongruities, a brief account of the discovery of the system prefaces the detailed description of the system itself. The biologically active products of complement activation and their effects are described in Chapter 2, and Chapter 3 details the dramatic recent developments in molecular biology which have greatly advanced our understanding of the complement system. The remaining chapters focus on the role of complement in diseases and the relevance of complement measurement to diagnosis and assessment of disease activity. As an aid to understanding the historical developments a simplified outline of the system is presented in Fig. 1.1.

## 2  The Complement System

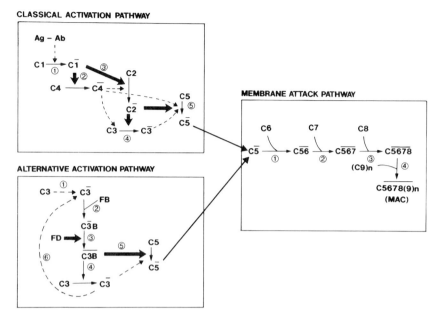

*Figure 1.1* The complement system, showing the division into three interacting pathways.

*The classical pathway:* (1) C1 activation; (2) C4 activation; (3) C2 activation; (4) C3 activation; (5) C5 activation.

*The alternative pathway:* (1) C3 activation; (2) Factor B binding; (3) Factor B cleavage; (4) C3 activation; (5) C5 activation.

*The membrane attack pathway:* (1) C56 formation (membrane); (2) C5–7 formation (fluid phase); (3) C5–8 formation (membrane); (4) MAC formation.

Enzymatic cleavages are represented by thick arrows and activated components or complexes are indicated by overlining.

### 1.2 HISTORICAL PERSPECTIVE

#### 1.2.1 Discovery of the system

In the late 19th century much scientific interest was focussed on the mechanisms by which the body defends itself against microorganisms. The predominant theory at that time was the Cellular Theory of Metchnikoff, who had demonstrated the presence in the blood of cells (phagocytes) which were capable of ingesting and destroying invading bacteria. A competing theory emerged from the work of Fodor, Nuttal, Buchner and others, who demonstrated a heat-labile bactericidal activity in fresh serum which Buchner termed *alexin* (Greek, *without a name*). Support for this 'humoral' theory of bacterolysis was provided by Jules Bordet, who examined the phenomenon (first described by Pfeiffer) of immune lysis of cholera vibrios and showed that here too the lytic factor was heat-labile. More importantly, Bordet demonstrated that immune lysis required two factors, a heat-stable factor present only in immune serum, which he termed *sensitizer*, and a heat-labile factor present also in nonimmune serum, which he considered to be identical to Buchner's alexin. Bordet then extended his studies of immune lysis to include the phenomenon of haemolysis of erythrocytes by immune serum. Here too he demonstrated the requirement for two factors, a heat-stable sensitizer (haemolysin) and a heat-labile alexin.

Meanwhile, Paul Ehrlich had been developing his 'side-chain' theory in an attempt to explain the appearance of *immune bodies* (antibodies) in immune serum. He examined erythrocyte haemolysis by immune serum and confirmed the requirement for two factors. The heat-stable factor he termed amboceptor or immune body, and the heat-labile factor, designated alexin by Buchner and Bordet, he called *complement* to indicate his opinion that this factor augmented or 'complemented' the haemolytic and bacterolytic properties inherent in the immune body. The terms alexin and complement were used interchangeably over the next 40 years to describe the labile lytic factor present in serum, and only in recent times has the former term fallen out of usage.

A vital concept to emerge from the work of Ehrlich was that of antibody and complement combining to form a complex enzyme capable of attacking and killing cells and microorganisms, antibody being the recognition unit and complement the catalytic site of the enzyme. Although the original concept envisaged the enzyme acting directly on the cell membrane, which we now know does not occur, the idea of a complex enzyme has endured and proven to be central to the functioning of complement.

Over the next few years an intense debate developed concerning the nature of complement and its interactions with antibodies, the main protagonists being Bordet and Ehrlich. Bordet's description of the 'complement fixation test' established that complement was involved quantitatively in immune haemolysis and was not merely an accessory factor as had been implied by Ehrlich in his choice of name, and enabled Robert Muir to provide the first meaningful definition of complement: *that labile substance of normal serum which is taken up by the combination of an antigen and its antisubstance.*

### 1.2.2 Elucidation of the components

The first indication that complement was not a single substance was provided by Ferrata. By dialysis of serum against water he separated serum proteins into two pools, the insoluble euglobulins and the soluble globulins. Complement haemolytic activity was absent both in the globulin fraction and in the resolubilized euglobulin pool. Recombination of the two restored lytic activity, demonstrating a requirement for at least two factors, one present in the euglobulin pool, which he termed 'midpiece', and the other a soluble globulin, termed 'endpiece'. These factors were subsequently renamed C'1 and C'2, respectively. Over the next 20 years application of the fractionation techniques available at that time by Coca, Whitehead and others allowed the definition of additional factors, named in order of their discovery C'3 and C'4.

Thus by the late 1920s at least four factors had been demonstrated to be required for the activity known as complement. The molecular nature of these factors was, however, completely unknown. Complement was still thought of as a serum lipoid or soap complex with the ability to dissolve membranes, or as a physicochemical state or colloidal attribute of fresh serum. Definitive evidence that the complement factors were proteins was not provided until the 1940s, when newly developed electrophoretic and ultracentrifugation techniques were applied to their purification. These techniques revealed that the factor C'3, described by Coca and by Whitehead in the 1920s, consisted of six proteins all involved in bringing about cell lysis. These proteins, initially termed C'3a–C'3f in order of their discovery, were purified and characterized by Nelson, Müller-Eberhard and their coworkers.

Around the same time the reaction sequence of the complement components was being unravelled, initially by Ueno and later by Mayer. Using partly purified components they showed that it was possible to *build up* the complement system sequentially on an antibody-sensitized erythrocyte, the first-acting component exposing or providing a binding site for the next component and so on. Formation of erythrocyte intermediates in this way enabled the reaction sequence to be defined. C'1 bound first followed sequentially by C'4, C'2, C'3a, C'3b, C'3e, C'3f, C'3c and C'3d. The terminology was simplified by the World Health Organization Committee on complement nomenclature in 1968, the new terminology being, in order of activation C1, C4, C2, C3, C5, C6, C7, C8 and C9.

### 1.2.3 The 'classical' activation pathway

Ehrlich had proposed that complement in combination with antibody functioned as an enzyme. Using erythrocyte intermediates produced by sequential addition of components as described above, Levine, Becker and others confirmed this hypothesis. Inhibitors of proteolytic enzymes prevented sequential activation and the intermediates themselves were capable of cleaving synthetic substrates. The nature of the enzymatic reactions remained unclear until the 1960s, when Mayer showed that activated C1 cleaved C2 into two fragments, C2a and C2b. The phenomenon of activation by enzymatic cleavage was shown to be of fundamental importance at all stages of the pathway, activation of C4, C3 and C5 requiring cleavage by specific enzymes or 'convertases' formed from the preceding components. From these studies the concept of an enzymatic cascade analogous to that occurring during coagulation emerged, the components being activated by cleavage in the order C1, C4, C2, C3, C5, the activation of each component creating a multimolecular complex capable of cleaving the next. The system became known as the 'classical' activation pathway, in order to distinguish it from alternative activation mechanisms described later. The reactions involved in activation are detailed in Section 1.3.1.

### 1.2.4 The alternative activation pathway

During the early years of this century it was noted by several workers that substances other than antibody could initiate activation of complement. Cobra venom and yeast cells were both shown to use up or consume complement when incubated with serum, indicating that activation was occurring. These early observations were extended in the 1940s by Pillemer and co-workers, who isolated the complement-activating substance zymosan from yeast cell walls. Pillemer showed that zymosan consumed C3 in a temperature- and magnesium-dependent manner, and that this activity required a serum factor which could be removed by prior incubation of serum with zymosan at low temperatures. He named this factor *properdin* from the Latin *perdere*, to lose or destroy. Serum depleted of properdin by adsorption with zymosan displayed decreased antibacterial and antiviral activity. A new complement system, termed the properdin system, was proposed, requiring properdin, complement and magnesium ions, together with a heat-labile factor (Factor B) and a hydrazine-sensitive factor (Factor A). The proposal provoked intense scientific and lay interest, stimulating many groups to begin investigations of the system. Alternative explanations of Pillemer's observations were suggested by several workers, notably Nelson, who demonstrated the existence of antibodies against zymosan in normal serum and suggested that activation of complement by these antibodies accounted for Pillemer's findings. In the wake of this controversy and with the death of Pillemer interest in the properdin system subsided. A further 10 years were to elapse before Pillemer's work was vindicated and the properdin system firmly established as a true alternative pathway of complement activation. Proof was provided by Lepow, who purified properdin to homogeneity and showed it to be capable of restoring bactericidal activity to zymosan-adsorbed serum, and by Gewurz and others, who showed that several known activators of complement, including endotoxin and zymosan, consumed large quantities of C3 and the late components without consuming the classical activation pathway components C1, C4 or C2. By the early 1970s the concept of an alternative complement activating pathway not requiring antibody but requiring properdin was fully established. Factor B was isolated by Lepow and shown to be distinct from the known complement proteins, but Factor A was found to be C3 of the classical pathway. A third protein component of the system, Factor D, was subsequently isolated by Müller-Eberhard and coworkers. The interactions of these proteins that occur during complement activation are discussed in Section 1.3.2.

### 1.2.5 The membrane attack pathway

One of the most remarkable properties of complement is its capacity to lyse cells, be they bacteria, erythrocytes or nucleated cells. By the early 1950s cell lysis was known to require 'classical' C'3, which contained C5, C6, C7, C8 and C9 in addition to C3, however, it was not clear which of these components were required for lysis. Then in the late 1960s Thompson, Lachmann and associates isolated a complex of activated C5 and C6 from acute phase serum and showed that it combined sequentially with C7, C8 and C9 to bring about cell lysis. This system, called 'reactive lysis', demonstrated that only these five proteins were required for cell lysis and that the activation pathway proteins did not participate directly.

The mechanisms by which complement caused cell lysis attracted much interest in the late 1950s. In a superb series of studies Green and Goldberg investigated tumor cell lysis and proposed that complement disrupted the cell membrane by forming holes through which small molecules could pass unimpeded. This concept was difficult to reconcile with the rigid concepts of membrane structure then current. Others reasoned that complement might acquire a detergent- or phospholipase-like activity on activation, thereby degrading the membrane, and this model was favoured until the early 1970s. By this time several pieces of data had accumulated: Borsos had shown by electron microscopy the presence on complement-lysed membranes of circular lesions; Lachmann had defined the protein requirements for complement lysis; Mayer had shown kinetically that a single active complex was sufficient to cause erythrocyte lysis; and Singer and Nicolson had proposed their fluid mosaic model which envisaged the membrane as an 'ordered fluid'. In the light of these observations Mayer in 1972 hypothesized that complement caused membrane damage by the formation of rigid channels in the cell membrane, as proposed earlier by Green and Goldberg. He suggested that the five complement proteins C5–C9 became inserted into the membrane following activation and formed a hollow transmembrane structure with a rigid central pore through which ions and water could pass. Experimental support for this *doughnut hypothesis* rapidly followed. The terminal components were shown to express hydrophobic sites on activation and to insert into the lipid bilayer, and the size of the membrane pore was defined. Although much debate has centred on the exact mechanism by which the terminal components bring about lysis and on the molecular composition of the lytic *membrane attack complex*, the basic concepts of Mayer's doughnut hypothesis have withstood the test of time. Current views on the formation, structure and mechanism of action of the membrane attack complex are detailed in Section 1.3.3.

### 1.2.6 Inflammation and opsonisation

Freiberg in 1910 demonstrated that immunization of guinea pigs with immune-complex-treated serum caused anaphylaxis. Heat inactivation of serum prevented anaphylaxis, leading several workers to conclude that the activity was derived from complement. Abundant evidence for this *humoral theory of anaphylaxis* was accumulated by Freiberg over the next 20 years but, despite this, complement-derived anaphylatoxins were not widely accepted as important mediators of inflammation. In the early 1960s Boyden demonstrated that incubation of fresh serum with immune complexes generated not only anaphylatoxin but also a chemotactic factor which attracted neutrophils. He suggested that this factor was also complement-derived. Proof of the origins of these active factors was soon provided by Müller-Eberhard and coworkers, who showed

8   *The Complement System*

that they were small fragments of C3 and C5 released by enzymatic cleavage during complement activation.

In the early years of this century it was recognized that incubation with serum rendered bacteria more easily ingested by phagocytic cells. This property of serum was shown to be heat-labile and consequently was thought to be complement-derived. Wright in 1904 coined the term *opsonification* to describe this property, meaning *preparation for ingestion*. A similar activity was described by Duke and Wallace in 1930. They showed that erythrocytes from some but not all species bound to serum-opsonised trypanosomes. Nelson, in 1953, showed that this phenomenon of erythrocyte binding also occurred on a variety of bacteria after treatment with immune sera, and called the phenomenon *immune adherence*. He later demonstrated that complement activation up to C3 was sufficient to cause immune adherence and proposed the existence on erythrocytes of receptors for C3 bound to the bacterial surface. Evidence for the existence of C3 receptors on neutrophils and on platelets was provided by several workers in the late 1960s. It is now clear that there are at least nine distinct types of complement receptors on different cell types, each having specific binding requirements and functions. A detailed description of these important molecules is provided in Chapter 2.

The major milestones in the history of the complement system are summarized in Table 1.1.

### 1.3 THE COMPLEMENT SYSTEM

The complement system is composed of at least 25 proteins. Of these, 12 are directly involved in the pathways constituting the system, while the remainder function as essential regulators. The known component and control proteins of the system, together with their important characteristics, are listed in Table 1.2.

Activation of the system initiates a sequence of biochemical reactions, each component activating the next in a cascade fashion. This cascade mechanism allows considerable amplification to occur in the system, a small initiating signal stimulating the formation of large quantities of active products. An essential requirement for such an amplification system to exist *in vivo* is the existence of stringent control mechanisms.

Multiple inhibitory and control proteins influence virtually every stage of the complement system, preventing excessive activation and damage to host cells. The system, represented in the simplest

Table 1.1 Milestones in the history of complement.

| | |
|---|---|
| 1896–1890 | Fodor, Nuttall and Buchner demonstrate a bacterolytic activity in fresh serum which Buchner names 'alexin' |
| 1894 | Pfeiffer observes lysis of cholera vibrios injected into the peritoneal cavity of immune guinea pigs — the Pfeiffer phenomenon |
| 1895–1889 | Bordet shows that two serum factors are required for immune bacterolysis or haemolysis — a thermostable 'sensitizer' and a thermolabile 'alexin' |
| 1899 | Ehrlich applies his side-chain theory to immune haemolysis and names the heat-labile serum component 'complement' |
| 1901 | Bordet and Gengou demonstrate that complement is consumed during immune haemolysis |
| 1907–1926 | Ferrata, Coca, Ritz and Whitehead show that complement comprises at least four components |
| 1909 | Freiberg demonstrates complement-derived anaphylactic activity – the humoral theory of anaphylaxis |
| 1941 | Pillemer and Heidelberger confirm the protein nature of complement components |
| 1954 | Pillemer discovers the alternative pathway of complement activation |
| 1955–1956 | Lepow, Becker and Levine demonstrate that C1 is a serine esterase acting on C2 and C4 |
| 1957–1966 | Nelson and coworkers separate 'classical' C3 into six distinct proteins |
| 1958–1966 | Mayer and associates elucidate the sequence of complement activation; Mayer proposes the 'one-hit' hypothesis |
| 1961–1968 | Müller-Eberhard and colleagues purify each of the complement components to homogeneity |
| 1962 | Boyden describes a complement-derived chemotactic activity |
| 1970 | Thompson and Lachmann establish the reactive lysis system |

terms in Fig. 1.1, is divisible into three interacting pathways, the classical and alternative activation pathways and the membrane attack pathway. The end-product of each activation pathway is an enzyme capable of cleaving C5 (a C5 convertase), and the first component of the membrane attack pathway is cleaved C5. The three interacting pathways will be described separately.

### 1.3.1 The classical activation pathway

The classical pathway, initiated by antigen–antibody complexes, consists of four plasma proteins, C1, C4, C2 and C3. C1 is made up

## The Complement System

Table 1.2 The proteins of the human complement system.

| | Component | Molecular weight (kDa) | Subunit structure | Plasma concentration mg/L | Plasma concentration (µM) | Role |
|---|---|---|---|---|---|---|
| Classical pathway | C1q | 460 | 6A chains (26 kDa), 6B chains (26 kDa), 6C chains (24 kDa) | 80 | (0.15) | Binds Ig; initiates classical pathway activation |
| | C1r | 83 | Single, complex with C1q | 50 | (0.30) | Cleaves/activates C1s |
| | C1s | 83 | In plasma (C1qC1r$_2$C1s$_2$) | 50 | (0.30) | Cleaves/activates C4 and C2 |
| | C4 | 205 | 1 α-chain (97 kDa), 1 β-chain (75 kDa), 1 γ-chain (33 kDa) | 600 | (3.0) | Binds C2 during activation |
| | C2 | 102 | Single chain | 20 | (0.20) | Cleaves/activates C3 and C5 |
| Alternative pathway | Factor B | 93 | Single chain | 210 | (2.0) | Cleaves/activates C3 and C5 |
| | Factor D | 24 | Single chain | 2 | (0.05) | Cleaves/activates Factor B |
| | Properdin | 220 | 4 identical subunits (55 kDa) | 26 | (0.10) | Stabilizes activation pathway convertases |
| Common | C3 | 185 | 1 α-chain (110 kDa); 1 β-chain (75 kDa) | 1300 | (7.0) | Binds C5 in convertases; opsonisation/chemotaxis, etc. |
| Membrane attack pathway | C5 | 190 | 1 α-chain (115 kDa); 1 β-chain (75 kDa) | 70 | (0.4) | Initiates membrane attack; C5a major chemotactic/anaphylactic peptide |
| | C6 | 120 | Single chain | 65 | (0.5) | |

# The Complement System

| | Component | MW (kDa) | Structure | Serum conc. μg/ml (μM) | Function |
|---|---|---|---|---|---|
| | C7 | 110 | Single chain | 55 (0.5) | Self-associate with cleaved C5 to form membrane sites to which C9 can bind |
| | C8 | 150 | 1 α-chain (64 kDa), 1 β-chain (64 kDa), 1 γ-chain (22 kDa) | 55 (0.4) | |
| | C9 | 69 | Single chain | 60 (0.8) | Major component of MAC |
| Soluble Control | C1-INH | 110 | Single chain | 200 (1.8) | Binds C1r+C1s, dissociates C1̄ |
| | C4bp | 500 | 8 identical subunits (70 kDa) | 250 (0.5) | Accelerates decay of C4b2a cofactor for C4b cleavage by I |
| | Factor H | 150 | Single chain | 450 (3.0) | Accelerates decay of C3bBb, cofactor for C3b cleavage by I; cleaves/inactivates C4b+C3b |
| | Factor I | 80 | 1 α-chain (50 kDa), 1 β-chain (38 kDa) | 35 (0.4) | |
| | S-protein | 83 | Single chain | 500 (6.0) | Binds fluid-phase C5b-7 |
| | Sp-40,40 | 70 | 2 subunits (35 kDa) | 50 | Binds fluid-phase C5b-7 |
| Membrane control | CR1 | 160–250 | Single chain | | Accelerate decay of C3/C5 convertases; cofactor in C3b cleavage |
| | DAF | 70 | Single chain | | |
| | MCP | 45–70 | Single chain | | |
| | HRF/MIP | 65 | Single chain | | Control of MAC formation/activity |
| | CD59 antigen | 20 | Single chain | | |

of three noncovalently linked subunits, C1q, C1r and C1s, association of which requires calcium ions. Because C1 assembly involves calcium, the classical activation pathway has an absolute requirement for this ion and is blocked in the presence of calcium chelators. The pathway is represented schematically in Fig. 1.2 and the different stages indicated.

#### 1.3.1.1 Recognition and C1 activation

The first component of complement, C1, is a large complex (total molecular weight about 800 kDa) composed of one molecule of C1q and two molecules each of C1r and C1s, association of the components requiring calcium ions. The recognition unit of the classical pathway, C1q, is a bizarre, multichain molecule containing a collagen-like stem portion from the end of which arise six globular 'heads', giving the appearance of a bunch of tulips (Fig. 1.3). C1q binds via its globular head regions to specific sites in the Fc region of the immunoglobulin molecule. Only IgG and IgM immunoglobulins

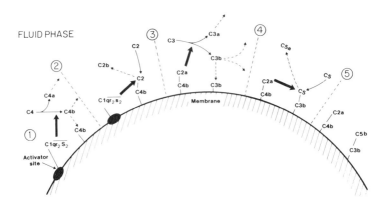

*Figure 1.2* The classical activation pathway.
*(1) C1 activation/C4 cleavage.* C1 binds to and is activated by antigens on the membrane. Activated C1 cleaves C4, releasing the small C4a fragment, C4b binding to the membrane close to C1. *(2) C2 cleavage.* C2 binds to C4b on the membrane and is cleaved by an adjacent C1, releasing a fragment C2b, C2a remaining bound to C4b. *(3) C3 cleavage.* C2a in the C4b2a complex cleaves C3, releasing C3a, the large fragment C3b binding to the membrane close to C4b2a. *(4) C5 binding and cleavage.* C5 binds to C3b on the membrane and is cleaved by C2a in an adjacent C4b2a complex, releasing a small fragment C5a. *(5) Initiation of membrane attack.* C5b, bound to C3b on the membrane, awaits binding of C6, the first step of the membrane attack pathway. Enzymatic cleavages are represented by thick arrows.

bind C1q and activate complement. Within the four subclasses of human IgG, $IgG_3$ is the most efficient binder of C1q, followed by $IgG_1$ and $IgG_2$. $IgG_4$ in most cases fails to bind C1q. For C1 activation to occur at least two of the six heads of C1q must interact with immunoglobulin. Because of its polyvalent structure a single IgM molecule can activate C1, but for IgG to initiate activation two molecules must be sufficiently close together on the target membrane or complex for the binding sites of a single C1q molecule to interact with both. Modelling of the C1q molecule based on electron micrographs indicates that the maximum distance it can span between adjacent IgG molecules is about 40 nm. Although binding to immunoglobulin remains the primary mechanism, it is becoming increasingly clear that other substances can bind and activate C1. Efficient activators include bacterial lipopolysaccharide, polyanionic compounds, viruses, C-reactive protein and myelin.

Binding of C1q to immunoglobulin (or other activators) initiates conformational changes within both C1q and C1r, resulting in the expression of neoantigens and the acquisition by C1r of esterolytic activity. Activated C1r cleaves the second C1r molecule in the $C1q(C1r)_2(C1s)_2$ complex, rendering it capable of cleaving and thereby activating C1s in the complex. The internal activation steps that occur during the activation of C1 are summarized in Fig. 1.3.

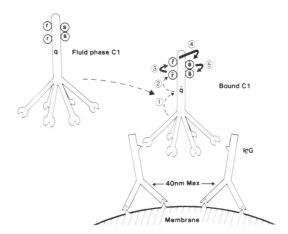

*Figure 1.3* Activation of C1.
C1, present in plasma as an inactive $C1q,r_2s_2$ complex, binds via at least two of its six 'arms' to immunoglobulin on the membrane. (*1*) binding causes conformational changes in C1q which result in its activation; (*2*) C1r activation by conformational change; (*3*) second C1r activated by enzymatic cleavage; (*4*) activated C1r cleaves and activates the first C1s which can then (*5*) cleave and activate the second C1s in the complex. Enzymatic cleavages are represented by thick arrows.

### 1.3.1.2 Cleavage of C4

The second stage in the classical pathway cascade involves the cleavage of C4 by C1. C4 is a molecule of about 200 kDa molecular weight which, though synthesized as a single polypeptide chain, is cleaved intracellularly into three chains (α, β and γ) held together by disulphide bonds. Activated C1s cleaves C4 at a single site in the α-chain, thereby releasing a 77 amino acid (8 kDa) N-terminal fragment, C4a, which is an anaphylatoxin (see Chapter 2). The larger fragment, C4b, acquires binding sites not expressed on the native molecule. Exposure of an internal thiolester group in the α-chain provides a site capable of interacting with membranes. This newly exposed membrane binding site allows covalent binding of C4b to surfaces by forming either ester linkages (binding to hydroxyl groups) or amide linkages (binding to amino groups). The site is extremely labile, having a lifetime of only a few microseconds. If C4b does not encounter a suitable surface during this time the site decays as a result of hydrolysis by surrounding water and the molecule is no longer able to bind. This lability makes C4b attachment a very inefficient process, only about 5% actually becoming bound to the surface, and also limits C4b deposition to a small area around the activating C1 complex. As a result, C4b binds in clusters within a radius of about 40 nm of the activating site. The intramolecular changes that occur during activation of C4 (and C3) are represented in Fig. 1.4.

### 1.3.1.3 Cleavage of C2

C2 is a single polypeptide chain of molecular weight 100 kDa. It is cleaved by activated C1 at a single site in the molecule into two fragments, C2a (73 kDa) and C2b (34 kDa). Cleavage of free C2 in solution by activated C1 on cells does not produce fragments capable of interacting with the cell surface or of participating further in the complement cascade. However, as well as its unstable membrane binding site, C4b possesses a stable site which binds C2 in the presence of magnesium ions. Although activated C1 can cleave free C2, the efficiency of cleavage is greatly enhanced when C2 is bound to an adjacent C4b molecule. Following cleavage the larger fragment, C2a, remains associated with C4b to form a C4b2a complex, the classical-pathway C3 convertase, which catalyses the next stage, cleavage of C3. The smaller fragment, C2b, may be released into the fluid phase where it has kinin activity (Chapter 2) or it may remain loosely attached to the C4b2a complex. The C4b2a complex is labile, with a lifetime of about one minute, decay

The Complement System 15

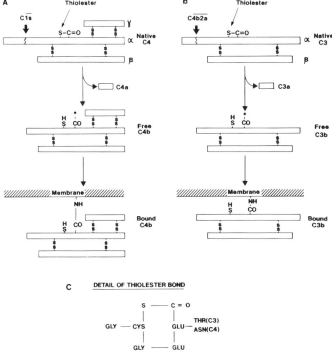

*Figure 1.4* Activation of C3 and C4.
The intramolecular changes that occur during the activation of C3 and C4 are very similar. (A) C4 is cleaved in its α-chain by C1s, releasing a small fragment and exposing a labile thiolester site in C4b which binds to amino or hydroxyl groups on the membrane. (B) C3 is similarly cleaved by C2a in the C4b2a complex, releasing a fragment and exposing the thiolester site. (C) Structure of the thiolester site of C4 and C3. Enzymatic cleavages are represented by thick arrows.

occurring as a result of dissociation of C2a. The controlling factors influencing this stage are described in Section 1.3.4.

#### 1.3.1.4 Cleavage of C3

C3 is a 190 kDa glycoprotein which, like C4 (with which it shares many structural and functional features), is synthesized as a single chain and post-translationally cleaved into two chains (α and β) held together by disulphide bonds. C3 is of central importance in the complement system. It is the complement protein present in the highest concentration in plasma (1.5 mg/l) and is involved in both the classical and alternative pathways. Cleavage of C3 by the C4b2a complex is in many ways analogous to C4 cleavage by activated C1. The catalytic site residing within C2a cleaves C3 in the fluid phase at a single point in the α-chain, releasing an N-terminal fragment, C3a

(77 amino acids, molecular weight 9 kDa), which is an important anaphylatoxin (Chapter 2). The large fragment, C3b, undergoes a conformational change, resulting in exposure of a labile thiolester site in the α-chain. As described above for C4b and illustrated in Fig. 1.4, this thiolester site can then bind covalently to hydroxyl or amino groups on target membranes. The short lifetime (about 60 μs) of the binding site restricts C3b fixation to the immediate vicinity of the C4b2a complex. Each C4b2a complex cleaves several hundred C3 molecules during its lifetime, but only about 10% of these bind to the cell via their labile membrane binding sites. The remaining molecules, which decay in the fluid phase to form the inactive product C3bi ('i' = inactive), take no further part in the complement cascade. They do, however, retain specific binding sites for complement receptors present on certain cell types, and binding of C3bi via these receptors is essential for the processes of opsonisation and phagocytosis described in Chapter 2. The molecular events involved in the activation, binding and decay of C3 are summarized in Fig. 1.5.

### 1.3.1.5 Cleavage of C5

The role of C3b in the continuation of the complement cascade is to provide a binding site for C5. Unlike C3, which is cleaved by the C4b2a complex in the fluid phase, C5 cannot be cleaved until after binding to C3b in the vicinity of the complex. C3b acts only as an acceptor for C5, rendering it susceptible to cleavage, but does not directly influence the enzymatic activity of C4b2a. Restriction of C5 activation in this way confines continued complement activation to the surface of the target cell.

C5 is a 190 kDa, two-chain protein structurally similar to C4 and C3. The C4b2a complex cleaves C5 at a single site in its α-chain, releasing a 74 amino acid N-terminal fragment, C5a, which has important anaphylactic and chemotactic properties (Chapter 2). The larger fragment, C5b, expresses labile binding sites not present on native C5, one of which allows C5b to bind weakly and reversibly to membranes (unlike C3 and C4, C5 does not possess a thiolester group) and the other of which binds C6. These binding sites are transient, with lifetimes of only a few minutes, but if C6 binds before decay of the membrane binding site, the site and hence the haemolytic potential of the complex is preserved.

Surprisingly, C5 can be activated *in vitro* without cleavage by exposure to acidic pH or by freeze-thawing in the presence of C6. The mechanisms by which these manipulations activate C5 are unclear but it is assumed that they cause transient conformational

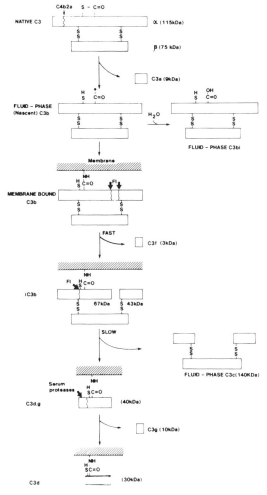

*Figure 1.5* Activation, binding and decay of C3.
Fluid-phase C3 is cleaved by C2a in the C4b2a complex to release the fragment C3a and expose the labile thiolester site on C3b. This site is prone to spontaneous hydrolysis, forming the inactive, fluid-phase C3bi. If C3b encounters a surface prior to decay of the thiolester it binds to hydroxyl or amino groups. Once bound to the surface, C3b is susceptible to the action of Factor I (FI), an enzyme which cleaves C3b at two sites in the α-chain, releasing a small fragment, C3f, and inactivating the molecule (iC3b). Factor I cleaves iC3b at another site in the α-chain, releasing the large fragment, C3c, leaving only the small C3d,g piece still attached to the surface. Nonspecific proteases further cleave this piece, releasing a fragment C3g, the 30 kDa C3d remaining on the surface. Enzymatic cleavages are represented by thick arrows.

changes in C5 similar to those caused by C4b2a-catalysed cleavage, exposing a membrane binding site and allowing C6 to bind. Even more surprising, perhaps, is the *in vitro* observation that in the presence of very high concentrations of C5, cleavage of C5 by the

C4b2a complex can occur in the absence of C3. The process is, however, very inefficient and is unlikely to be of relevance under normal conditions *in vivo*.

### 1.3.2 The alternative pathway

The alternative pathway of complement activation provides a nonspecific natural defence system against microorganisms and other pathogens which operates independently of specific antibody. This pathway is comprised of six plasma proteins, of which three are responsible for activation and amplification (C3, Factor B, Factor D), the other three (properdin, Factor H, Factor I) mediating control (see Table 1.1). The alternative pathway is active against a wide range of targets, including pathogenic microorganisms, virus-infected cells, neoplastic cells and erythrocytes from certain species. Phylogenetically it is an older system than the classical pathway, an activity analogous to the alternative pathway being present in sea urchins and other primitive animals which have no antibody-activated complement equivalent. The pathway is divisible into several distinct stages (Fig. 1.6).

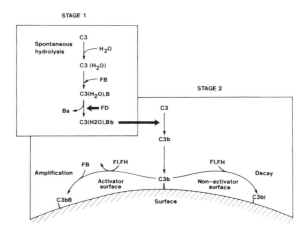

*Figure 1.6* The alternative activation pathway.
In the fluid phase (Stage 1), slow, spontaneous hydrolysis of C3 produces a molecule C3($H_2O$) capable of binding Factor B (FB) to form a soluble convertase which can cleave more C3. Small amounts of C3b are thus continually deposited on all surfaces (Stage 2). The outcome of this event depends on the nature of the surface. Activator surfaces protect C3b from inactivation by Factors H and I and favour binding of Factor B, forming bound C3/C5 convertases. Nonactivator surfaces allow Factors H and I ready access to bound C3b, resulting in rapid inactivation. Enzymatic cleavages are represented by thick arrows.

### 1.3.2.1 Formation of the initial C3 convertase

An essential component of the C3 convertase of the alternative pathway is cleaved C3 (C3b) itself (Fig. 1.6). This requirement poses an interesting conundrum which has attracted great research interest. If C3b is required for subsequent cleavage of C3, how is the first C3 molecule cleaved? Despite many attempts, no specific initiating factor has been found. The current concept, which is supported by recent experimental evidence, is that the alternative pathway is continuously undergoing low-grade spontaneous activation, the 'tick-over' hypothesis. When this hypothesis was first advanced it was thought that spontaneous activation was brought about by enzymatic cleavage of C3. It is now evident that no enzyme is involved, activation of C3 occurring as a result of spontaneous hydrolysis of its internal thiolester bond to form a molecule $C3(H_2O)$ which, apart from its inability to bind covalently to surfaces, is functionally equivalent to C3b. In the presence of magnesium ions, $C3(H_2O)$ binds Factor B in the fluid phase, rendering it susceptible to cleavage/activation by Factor D (see below) and thereby forming a fluid-phase C3 convertase $C3(H_2O),Bb(Mg)$.

### 1.3.2.2 Formation of membrane-bound C3 convertases

Factor B is a single-chain protein of molecular weight 93 kDa which is structurally and functionally homologous with C2 of the classical pathway. Upon binding to activated C3 it is rendered susceptible to cleavage by Factor D, a serine esterase present in its active state in the fluid phase. Cleavage of Factor B releases a 33 kDa fragment, Ba, which may have mitogenic activity. The Bb fragment, while bound to activated C3, has serine esterase activity and, like C2a, is capable of cleaving C3 and C5.

The spontaneously generated fluid-phase convertase $C3(H_2O),Bb(Mg)$ cleaves C3 in precisely the same way as the C4b2a complex of the classical pathway, releasing the anaphylatoxin C3a and exposing the thiolester binding site on C3b. C3b formed in this way binds to any surface it encounters during the lifetime of its binding site. Thus, C3b is deposited continuously in a random and nonspecific way on the surfaces of host cells and pathogenic organisms alike. Whether activation of the pathway continues is determined by properties of the surface. C3b bound to nonactivating surfaces (e.g. host cells) is rapidly inactivated by the control proteins Factors H and I, whereas C3b bound to activating surfaces is protected from these factors and therefore persists. Specifically, it appears that C3b on activating surfaces is not accessible to Factor H, which cannot therefore bind and accelerate inactivation. The properties of a surface which allow alternative pathway activation to occur are still not fully resolved, but surfaces rich in carbohydrate and deficient in sialic acid tend to be the best activators. Absence of sialic acid may be of particular importance as its removal from cells which are normally resistant to alternative pathway activation can render them vulnerable.

### 1.3.2.3 Amplification on activator surfaces

C3b on the cell surface binds Factor B in the presence of magnesium ions, thereby rendering it susceptible to cleavage/activation by Factor D. The bound C3b,Bb(Mg) complex can then cleave more C3, initiating a positive feedback cycle which rapidly amplifies the amount of C3b present on the cell surface, generating large amounts of anaphylatoxin in the process (Fig. 1.7). Control of such a potentially explosive cycle must be strict. This is achieved by the spontaneous decay of the C3b,Bb(Mg) complex (lifetime about 2 minutes), and by the action of the control proteins described in Section 1.3.4.

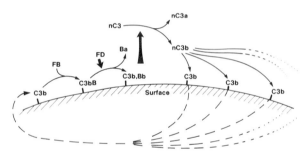

*Figure 1.7* Amplification in the alternative pathway.
On an activating surface, bound C3b is protected from inactivators and binds Factor B to form a C3b,Bb complex. This complex cleaves more C3, resulting in the deposition of large amounts of C3b on the surface. Each newly deposited C3b is itself capable of binding Factor B thus forming a new C3 convertase, resulting in rapid amplification. Enzymatic cleavages are represented by thick arrows.

### 1.3.2.4 Cleavage of C5

Binding of a second C3b molecule in the immediate vicinity of a C3b,Bb(Mg) complex results in the formation of the alternative-pathway C5 convertase. The events are analogous to C5 cleavage in the classical pathway. C3b binds C5 and presents it to the adjacent C3b,Bb(Mg) complex (C4b2a in the classical pathway) in the appropriate conformation for cleavage by Bb (C2a in the classical pathway). Cleavage results in release of the anaphylatoxin C5a, and exposes membrane- and C6-binding sites on the large fragment, C5b.

## 1.3.3 The membrane attack pathway

Cleavage of C5 by the convertase of either the classical or alternative activation pathways is the final enzymatic step in the complement cascade. The membrane attack pathway, which begins with the formation of C5b, proceeds via the sequential assembly of C5b, C6, C7, C8 and C9 into a heteropolymeric complex with the capacity to insert into and damage cell membranes, the membrane attack complex (MAC). As described above, C5 cleavage occurs almost exclusively on the surface of the target cell, thereby restricting membrane attack to that cell. The events that occur at the cell membrane during MAC assembly are summarized in Fig. 1.8.

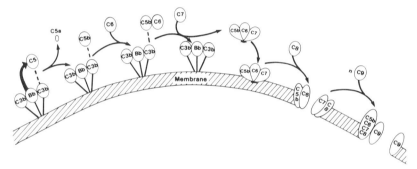

*Figure 1.8* The membrane attack pathway.
C5 is cleaved by the C5 convertase of either the classical or alternative pathways. The large fragment, C5b, remains attached to C3b in the convertase, and binds C6 from the fluid phase. Binding of C7 to the C5b6 complex causes its release from the C5 convertase and the acquisition of a labile membrane binding site through which the C5b67 complex attaches directly to the membrane but does not disturb membrane integrity. Binding of C8 to this complex results in deeper penetration into, and some disruption of, the membrane. Multiple molecules of C9 are then incorporated into the complex to form the complete membrane attack complex.

### 1.3.3.1 Assembly of the membrane attack complex (MAC)

Newly formed C5b, still bound to its convertase, expresses transient binding sites for membranes and for C6, a single-chain glycoprotein of 110 kDa molecular weight. If C6 does not bind to C5b during the lifetime of its binding site (about 2 minutes), both sites decay and C5b is no longer active. Binding of C6 creates a stable complex with weak membrane binding properties and the capacity to bind C7, a single-chain glycoprotein of 110 kDa which is structurally similar to C6. The complex may be released from the convertase at the C5b6 stage but usually remains attached until after C7 has bound. Binding of C7 causes major conformational changes in the complex, effecting its release from the C5 convertase and exposing a transient hydrophobic membrane binding site. If the C5b67 complex does not rapidly encounter a membrane it self-aggregates and interacts with inhibitory proteins in the fluid phase, and consequently the binding site is lost. Deposition of C5b67 is thus restricted to the target cell. A small proportion of complexes may become deposited on host cells in close proximity to the target, damaging or destroying them — the phenomenon of *innocent bystander lysis*. Once membrane-bound, the C5b67 complex is stable and resistant to removal from the cell surface. Although there is evidence that this complex inserts into the lipid bilayer of the membrane, it causes little disturbance of membrane structure and does not damage the cell.

The fourth component of the MAC, C8, is a 150 kDa glycoprotein with a very unusual three-chain structure. The $\alpha$- and $\gamma$-chains are disulphide-linked, whereas the $\beta$-chain is noncovalently bound in the complex. C8 binds to C5b in the C5b67 complex via a binding site in the C8 $\beta$-chain. The $\alpha$-chain of C8 is responsible for binding the final component of the MAC, C9. The role of the C8 $\gamma$-chain is as yet uncertain. It is not required for lytic activity, as C8 containing only the $\alpha$- and $\beta$-chains retains full haemolytic potential. Incorporation of C8 into the C5b67 complex causes the complex to become more deeply embedded in the membrane, making it slightly leaky. The leak caused by the C5b–8 complex may be sufficient to cause slow lysis of metabolically inert targets, such as aged sheep erythrocytes, but actively metabolizing cells, by virtue of their ion pumps, are able to resist lysis. Binding of C9 to the complex greatly enhances membrane perturbation.

C9 is a 69 kDa single-chain glycoprotein present in plasma in a globular hydrophilic form. Binding of C9 to the $\alpha$-chain of C8 initiates major conformational changes in C9 allowing it to insert deeply into the membrane, greatly enhancing the lytic activity of the MAC.

### 1.3.3.2 MAC structure and C9 polymerization

When erythrocytes lysed by complement are viewed under the electron microscope numerous cylindrical structures are seen on the membrane. These cylinders are remarkably homogeneous: viewed from above they have the appearance of rings with an outer diameter of 20 nm surrounding a 'pore' of 10 nm diameter, and in side view they are elongated structures about 16 nm in height which insert deeply into the membrane (Fig. 1.9). Abundant evidence now exists that these structures represent the MAC, but the exact

## The Complement System   23

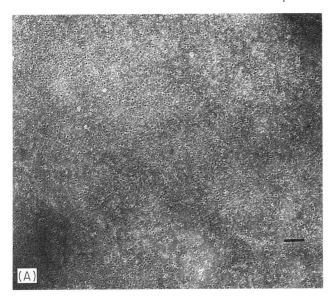

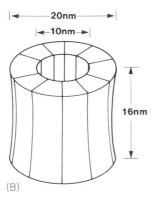

*Figure 1.9* Membrane attack complex (MAC) structure.
(A) Electron micrograph of a sheep erythrocyte lysed with human complement and negatively stained with uranyl acetate. The membrane is covered with ring lesions having a central 'pore' of 10 nm diameter. The scale bar represents 100 nm. (B) Schematic representation of the MAC based on electron-microscopic evidence. The MAC is envisaged as a hollow cylinder formed from the component proteins of the membrane attack pathway which inserts into and traverses the membrane. Electron micrograph kindly provided by Dr J. R. Dankert, University of Florida.

composition of the complex has attracted much debate. The early models envisaged the MAC tubule being assembled like a barrel, each of the five component proteins providing one stave of the barrel. In order to account for the apparent size of the complex a dimeric structure was suggested, each set of five proteins forming half the barrel. An alternative hypothesis was that C9 alone was present in multiple copies, the complex having the structure C5b678(9)$_n$, where $n$ was any number from 1 to 12. Addition of C9 'staves' in this way also provided an explanation of the observed size heterogeneity of the functional pores formed by the MAC (Fig. 1.10).

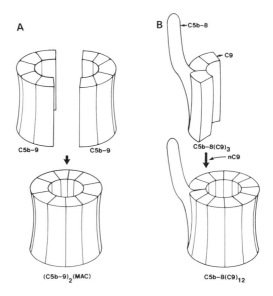

*Figure 1.10* Models of membrane attack complex (MAC) assembly.
(A) *C5b–9 dimer model.* In this model, now disproven, the MAC is constructed from two C5b–9 complexes, each complex forming half of the cylinder, and all component proteins contributing to the walls of the cylinder. (B) *Poly-C9 model.* In this more recent model, the components C5b–8 have little or no involvement in the final structure of the MAC cylinder but occupy a peripheral position, the cylinder walls being formed by up to 12 C9 molecules.

This latter hypothesis has received considerable support from studies on the behaviour of isolated C9. Incubation of pure C9 at low ionic strength or in the presence of zinc ions causes spontaneous polymerization with the formation of tubular structures containing between 12 and 18 molecules of C9, which are almost

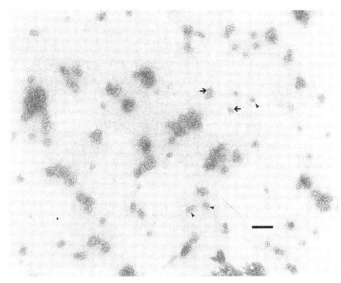

*Figure 1.11* Electron micrograph of poly-C9.
Pure C9 polymerized in the presence of zinc ions. The tubular structures seen both in side view (arrows) and 'head on' (arrowheads) are virtually indistiguishable from the membrane attack complex formed on erythrocyte membranes. The scale bar represents 100 nm. Electron micrograph kindly provided by Dr J. R. Dankert, University of Florida.

indistinguishable from the structures seen on complement-lysed membranes (Fig. 1.11). It was therefore suggested that the tubular membrane lesion consists entirely of polymerized C9, the C5b–8 complex functioning to catalyse polymerization but having no direct role in the formation of the lesion (Fig. 1.10). During polymerization C9 undergoes considerable conformational change, the globular, hydrophilic monomer unfolding into an elongated conformation with the capacity to self-associate and insert into membranes.

Although this is currently the most accepted model of MAC structure several anomalies remain. A complex containing a single C9 molecule is capable of causing cell lysis, and C9 which has been proteolytically modified to prevent ring polymer formation retains full lytic activity. The relevance of ring polymer formation by C9, and the tubular membrane structure for which it is undoubtedly responsible, to the lytic action of the MAC therefore remains controversial.

### 1.3.3.3 Cell lysis by the MAC

Irrespective of the exact structure of the lytic MAC it is clear that the complex does form functional pores in the membrane through which ions and small molecules can pass. C9 in the MAC completely traverses the membrane, being exposed at the external and cytoplasmic faces. Rigid, protein-lined pores may exist at the centre of the MAC, but such a structure is not necessary for the formation of stable transmembrane channels and is difficult to reconcile with the known pore size heterogeneity. Insertion of C9 through the membrane will cause disturbances in the surrounding lipid and hence formation of a functional pore alongside the inserted molecule. Addition of more C9 will increase lipid disturbance, thereby increasing the size of the functional pore.

Because of the high intracellular osmotic pressure, formation of a transmembrane channel in the normally impermeant membrane bilayer allows water, ions and small molecules to flow into the cell, causing cell swelling and, in the case of metabolically inert targets, cell lysis — the process of colloid osmotic lysis. A single functional channel is sufficient to cause lysis of an aged erythrocyte. Lysis of metabolically active target cells is, however, much less efficient.

Several fluid-phase and membrane-associated inhibitors of MAC function exist and are described in Section 1.3.4.

### 1.3.3.4 Membrane attack on nucleated cells

The favoured targets for studies of MAC action have been erythrocytes and liposomes. These inert targets have proved useful in determining how the MAC interacts with membranes, but their relevance to the role of the MAC *in vivo*, where the target cells are by and large metabolically active and nucleated, is limited. Nucleated cells are much more difficult to kill with the MAC than are erythrocytes. Many thousands of complexes can be deposited on a cell without lysis. Two major factors limit lysis of nucleated cells: firstly, ion pumps counteract the influx of ions and water through the MAC pores, minimizing cell swelling; and secondly, active recovery processes rapidly remove MACs from the cell surface by endocytosis or exocytosis (Fig. 1.12). Nucleated cells can therefore

---

*Figure 1.12* Resistance of nucleated cells to MAC lysis.
Nucleated cells, by virtue of nonspecific and specific resistance mechanisms, are able to withstand limited complement membrane attack. (*A*), (*B*) Scanning electron micrographs of human neutrophils prior to or during nonlethal complement attack. During attack vesicular projections appear on the cell surface from which MAC-rich vesicles are shed. (*C*) Schematic representation of resistance mechanisms in nucleated cells. Ions and water entering the cell via the MAC are removed by energy-consuming ion pumps. MACs are also physically removed from the cell surface by endocytosis and/or exocytosis, the stimuli for which may include increased intracellular calcium concentration. Lysis occurs only when energy stores are empty or when the rate of formation of MACs exceeds the capacity of the cell to remove them.

The Complement System 27

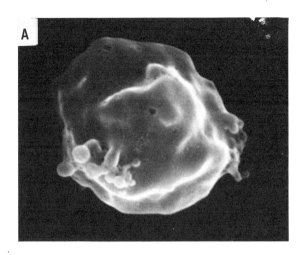

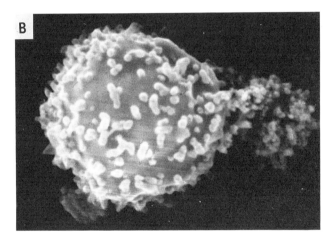

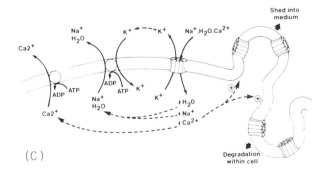

survive limited membrane attack. Nevertheless, membrane attack may profoundly affect cell function. Some of these nonlethal effects are described in Chapter 2.

### 1.3.3.5 Similarities between the MAC and T-cell perforins

Cytotoxic T cells (CTLs) and natural killer (NK) cells bring about target cell lysis by releasing the contents of their cytoplasmic granules into the intercellular space (Fig. 1.13). These granules contain protein molecules which are toxic to the target cell. One of the granule toxins is a protein of about 65 kDa molecular weight, called perforin. This protein has been isolated and shown to be capable of causing cell lysis in the absence of other granule constituents by, in the presence of calcium ions, inserting into the target cell membrane and forming transmembrane pores. In the membrane, perforin self-polymerizes to form lesions which under the electron microscope appear remarkably similar to the MAC (Fig. 1.13). Perforin also self-polymerizes in a calcium-dependent manner in the absence of membranes to form ring polymers of similar dimensions to poly-C9. These functional and structural similarities have led to the suggestion that perforin represents a primitive, non-targeted lytic system out of which the multicomponent, targeted MAC has evolved. How the perforin-producing cell avoids lysis by its own products remains an intriguing puzzle.

### 1.3.4 Control of the complement system

At each stage of complement activation control is achieved by a combination of two factors: firstly, the spontaneous decay of the active factor; and secondly, the influence of specific regulatory proteins which accelerate (or occasionally slow) this natural decay process. The following sections detail the proteins involved in control, but the importance of spontaneous decay of activity throughout the system should be borne in mind.

#### 1.3.4.1 Control in the classical activation pathway

Control at the stage of C1 activation is mediated by *C1 inhibitor* (C1-INH), the only naturally occurring inhibitor of the two proteases of C1 (C1r and C1s). C1-INH is a serum glycoprotein with a molecular weight of about 100 kDa which not only regulates C1 activation but also inhibits enzymes of the clotting, kallikrein and plasmin systems. It is an extremely efficient inhibitor, restricting the half-life of activated C1 to only about 20 seconds at physiological concentra-

The Complement System 29

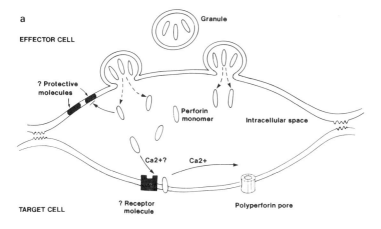

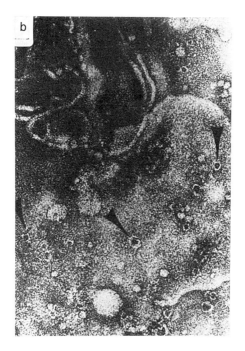

*Figure 1.13* Perforin-mediated cell lysis.
(*a*) Perforins are present in the granules of natural killer or cytotoxic T cells (effector). Upon binding of the effector cell to the target, perforin molecules are released into the intercellular space and bind to the target cell membrane. In the presence of calcium, polymerization of perforin occurs in the membrane to form cylindrical structures similar in appearance to the MACs which bring about target lysis. The factors which protect the effector cell from autolysis remain unknown. (*b*) Electron micrograph of an erythrocyte lysed by perforin. The membrane is covered with ring lesions (arrowed) with an internal diameter of about 8 nm. Electron micrograph from Podack and Konigsberg, *J. Exp. Med.* **160**, 695 (1984), with permission.

tions. It also functions to restrict autoactivation of fluid-phase C1, probably by loosely combining with the molecule in plasma. Genetic deficiency of C1-INH causes the disease known as hereditary angioedema, described in detail in Chapter 4. Inhibition of activated C1 involves the covalent binding of C1-INH to the catalytic sites on C1r and C1s, followed by dissociation of these molecules from C1q. The dissociated complex contains one molecule each of C1r and C1s and two molecules of C1-INH. Measurement of this complex in plasma can provide evidence of classical pathway activation *in vivo* (see Chapter 12).

Several proteins are involved in control at the stage of assembly and decay of the C4b2a complex. *C4 binding protein* (C4bp) is a large plasma protein (molecular weight 500 kDa, seven identical chains) which can bind up to six molecules of C4b. Binding of C4bp blocks the C2 combining site, preventing further interaction of C4b with C2. It thereby directly accelerates dissociation of the C4b2a complex and also serves as a cofactor for the enzymes responsible for C4b cleavage (see below). Two membrane proteins also act as cofactors for C4b cleavage enzymes. The C3 receptor $CR_1$, present on erythrocytes and leucocytes, binds C4b alone or in the convertase and enhances its cleavage. *Membrane cofactor protein* (MCP), as its name implies, also serves as a cofactor for C4b cleavage. It is a rather heterogeneous membrane protein (molecular weight range 45–70 kDa) which binds C4b and enhances its cleavage. *Decay accelerating factor* (DAF) is a 70 kDa protein present on the membranes of erythrocytes, platelets, leucocytes and epithelial cells. It acts in a similar way to C4bp, causing dissociation of the C4b2a complex, but does not act as a cofactor for C4b cleavage. It may also bind C4b alone, thereby preventing convertase formation. Cleavage of C4b, the second stage in C3 convertase inactivation, is catalysed by *Factor I* a fluid-phase serine protease. This enzyme, in the presence of any of the cofactors C4bp, MCP or $CR_1$, cleaves C4b at two sites in the molecule, releasing a large fragment, C4c, the small C4d fragment remaining attached to the membrane.

Control at the level of the C5 convertase utilizes the same factors. C4bp and DAF accelerate dissociation of the complex, and Factor I, in concert with its cofactors C4bp, $CR_1$ and MCP, cleaves C3b. Factor I cleaves C3b at two sites in the α-chain, releasing a small fragment, C3f, and in the process inactivating the molecule. On erythrocytes, further cleavage of the inactivated C3b (iC3b) by Factor I occurs, releasing a large fragment, C3c, while a smaller piece, C3dg, remains attached to the membrane. The stages involved in the inactivation of C4b and C3b are illustrated in Fig. 1.14.

*The Complement System* 31

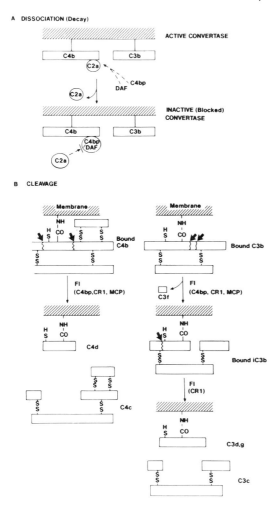

*Figure 1.14* Control of the classical-pathway C3 convertase.
Inactivation of the C4b2a complex involves two processes. (*A*) Dissociation of C2a from the bound C4b occurs spontaneously but is greatly accelerated by the membrane protein decay accelerating factor (DAF) or by the serum C4 binding protein (C4bp). Binding of these proteins to C4b also blocks subsequent rebinding of C2a. (*B*) Cleavage of bound C4b is mediated by Factor I (FI) in the presence of one of several cofactors: C4bp, $CR_1$ or MCP. FI cuts C4b at two sites in the α-chain, releasing a large fragment, C4c, and leaving the small C4d piece attached to the membrane. Cleavage of C4b closely resembles that of C3b. Thick arrows represent proteolytic cleavages.

### 1.3.4.2 Control in the alternative activation system

Many of the controlling factors operating in the classical activation pathway also modulate activation in the alternative pathway. Thus, both $CR_1$ and DAF accelerate decay of the alternative-pathway C3

## 32 The Complement System

and C5 convertases (C3b,Bb and C3b,Bb,C3b, respectively), $CR_1$ by binding C3b and DAF by binding Factor B. Factor I inactivates the convertases by cleavage of C3b but requires a cofactor distinct from those operative in the classical pathway. This protein, *Factor H*, binds to C3b in the convertases and competes for the Factor B

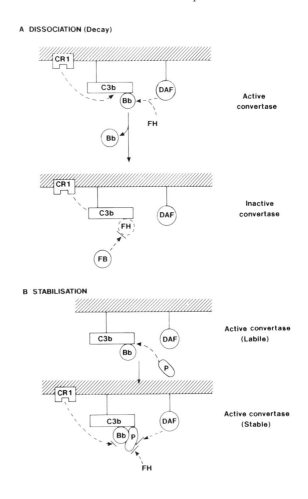

*Figure 1.15* Control of the alternative pathway C3 convertase.
The C3b,Bb complex, which undergoes slow, spontaneous dissociation, is subject to both positive and negative control. (A) Negative control is mediated by factors which accelerate the spontaneous dissociation of the complex, the membrane proteins decay accelerating factor (DAF) and complement receptor 1 ($CR_1$), and the serum protein Factor H (FH). FH also prevents reassembly of the complex by binding to C3b and blocking the binding of Factor B (FB). (B) Positive control or stabilization occurs when the serum protein properdin (P) binds to the C3b,Bb complex. Binding of properdin protects the complex from the decay-enhancing factors noted above, prolonging the lifetime of the complex.

binding site. Consequently it accelerates dissociation of the complex as well as allowing cleavage by Factor I to occur. Factor H also competes with C5 for binding to C3b in the C5 convertase, further inhibiting C5 activation.

The other control protein unique to the alternative pathway is *properdin*, a large (224 kDa), highly basic protein present in plasma in an inactive form. Properdin is activated upon binding to C3b and stabilizes the alternative-pathway C3 and C5 convertases. The effect of properdin is therefore the converse of that of Factor H (Fig. 1.15).

### 1.3.4.3 Control in the membrane attack pathway

Formation of the potentially cytolytic membrane attack complex is strictly regulated. Until very recently regulation was thought to be mediated solely by fluid-phase inhibitors. The recent demonstration of membrane proteins which also modulate MAC activity has altered our perception of MAC control.

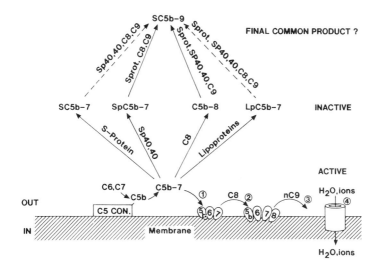

*Figure 1.16* Control of membrane attack complex (MAC) formation.
MAC formation is controlled by membrane-associated and fluid-phase factors. In the fluid phase the C5b–7 complex may encounter one of several inhibitors, S-protein, Sp-40,40, C8 or lipoprotein. Binding of any of these proteins will block the membrane binding site, rendering the complex inactive. Subsequent binding of C8 and C9, and perhaps the other inhibitors, results in the formation of the fluid-phase SC5b–9 complex. Once C5b–7 is bound to the membrane it is protected from the action of fluid-phase inhibitors, but on homologous cells, is controlled by membrane MAC inhibitors. The stage at which these proteins influence MAC function remains to be established — whether by inhibiting C5b–7 binding (*1*), binding of C8 (*2*), binding of C9 (*3*), or formation of the pore (*4*).

Regulation in the fluid phase prevents the spread of MACs from the site of activation, restricting effects to the target cell. The major fluid-phase inhibitor of the MAC is *S-protein*, an acidic glycoprotein with a molecular weight of about 80 kDa. S-protein binds to fluid-phase C5b–7 complexes at a site close to the membrane-binding site, forming an SC5b–7 complex and preventing interaction with membranes. C8 and C9 subsequently bind to the SC5b–7 complex to form a cytolytically inactive fluid-phase SC5b–9 complex containing three molecules of S-protein, two or three molecules of C9 and one molecule each of the other terminal components. A novel serum protein, SP–40,40, has recently been described which inhibits MAC formation in a similar manner to S-protein and is incorporated into the SC5b–9 complex. Binding of the nascent C5b–7 complex to membranes is also inhibited in a nonspecific fashion by all types of serum lipoproteins, which compete for the membrane binding site of the C5b–7 complex. C8 itself can also be considered to be a fluid-phase inhibitor of MAC formation, binding of C8 to fluid-phase C5b–7 rendering it incapable of subsequent membrane binding.

Regulation of MAC formation and activity on the membrane is mediated by a recently discovered group of MAC-inhibiting proteins. Two types of proteins have been described, one with a molecular weight of about 65 kDa and the other of about 20 kDa. They are present on erythrocytes, platelets and leucocytes. The mechanisms by which these proteins inhibit MAC function and their importance in the protection of host cells *in vivo* have yet to be established. Control of MAC formation and activity is summarized in Fig. 1.16.

## 1.4 FURTHER READING

*Historical*

Bouldan, C. (1910). *Collected Studies in Immunity*. Wiley, New York. (A collection of landmark papers in immunology from the 1890s and early 1900s. Includes the important studies of Paul Ehrlich.)

Mayer, M. M. (1984). Complement: historical perspectives and some current issues. *Complement* **1**, 2–26. (A brief but well-referenced history of the complement system.)

*The classical pathway*

Loos M. (1988). 'Classical' pathway of activation. In: Rother, K. and Till, G. O. (eds), *The Complement System*. Springer, Berlin, pp. 136–154.

Hughes-Jones, N. (1986). The classical pathway. In: Ross, G. D. (ed.), *Immunobiology of the Complement System*. Academic Press, New York, pp. 21–44.

*The alternative pathway*

Pangburn, M. K. and Müller-Eberhard, H. J. (1984). The alternative pathway of complement. *Springer Semin. Immunopathol.* **7**, 163–192. (An excellent review with over 150 references.)

*The membrane attack pathway*

Esser, A. F. (1982). Interactions between complement proteins and biological and model membranes. In: Chapman, D. (ed.), *Biological Membranes. Vol. 4*. Academic Press, New York, pp. 277–325.

Podack, E. R. (1988). Assembly and structure of the membrane attack complex (MAC) of complement. In: Podack, E. R. (ed.), *Cytolytic Lymphocytes and Complement: Effectors of the Immune System. Vol. 1*. CRC Press, Boca Raton, Florida, pp. 173–184.

Morgan, B. P. (1989). Complement membrane attack on nucleated cells: resistance, recovery and non-lethal effects. *Biochem. J.* **264**, 1–14. (A review of modern concepts of MAC action containing 157 references.)

CHAPTER TWO
# The Biological Effects of Complement Activation

## 2.1 INTRODUCTION

Activation of the complement system results in the production of molecules with potent biological activities. Fragments with anaphylactic and chemotactic activities and with the capacity to enhance elimination of foreign particles are generated, and the final product, the membrane attack complex (MAC), can kill or stimulate the cells on which it is formed. In this chapter the factors responsible for each of these activities are described. In most cases, production of the biological effect requires interaction of complement fragments with specific receptors present on cells. The varieties and functions of these *complement receptors* are also discussed here.

## 2.2 PRO-INFLAMMATORY EFFECTS OF COMPLEMENT ACTIVATION

At any site of tissue injury in the body, whether traumatic, chemical or infective, an inflammatory reaction occurs. This is characterized by localized vasodilatation and increased capillary permeability, resulting in leakage of fluid into the site, and by migration of phagocytic cells into the area. At the inflammatory site well-recognized signs and symptoms occur including swelling (due to fluid leakage into the tissues), heat and redness (due to increased capillary blood flow). Complement activation at the site of injury is a major mediator of these effects. Activation occurs on the surfaces of invading microorganisms and on damaged tissue, releasing from the focus of inflammation complement fragments which directly and indirectly aid the destruction of the inflammatory stimulus.

## 2.2.1 The anaphylactic factors

Encounters with certain antigens can lead, in sensitive individuals, to an immediate tissue reaction occurring within minutes of antigen combining with antibody. The reaction, known as anaphylaxis, is caused by the release of histamine and other active molecules from mast cells in the tissues. Anaphylaxis may be localized to specific organs or may be generalized, resulting in shock. Classically, anaphylaxis follows binding of antigen to antibody (usually IgE) on the mast cell surface. Complement-derived factors can also stimulate the release of active products from mast cells, thereby stimulating anaphylaxis.

The complement proteins C4, C3 and C5 are closely related structurally and during activation each is cleaved in a similar fashion, releasing peptides of about 70–80 amino acids from the N-terminal ends of their α-chains. In each case cleavage by the appropriate convertase occurs at an arginyl–X–peptide bond, the resultant peptides all having C-terminal arginine residues. These anaphylactic peptides, C4a, C3a and C5a, are structurally and functionally alike but differ in their relative potency. C5a is by far the most efficient anaphylactic agent, followed by C3a, C4a having only weak activity (Table 2.1). Control of anaphylactic peptide activity is achieved efficiently *in vivo* by the presence in plasma of an enzyme, *carboxypeptidase N*, which acts as an anaphylatoxin inactivator. This enzyme removes the C-terminal arginine residue from each peptide. The *desArg* (minus arginine) derivatives thus formed are, with the exception of C5a desArg, completely inactive. C5a desArg, although about 2000-fold less potent than C5a, retains anaphylactic activity and is stable. Unlike the other anaphylactic peptides it is therefore able to diffuse from the site of inflammation and cause more widespread effects. C5a is the most active of the anaphylactic peptides in its native form, the most resistant to cleavage by carboxypeptidase N, and its cleavage product C5a desArg retains some biological activity. It is therefore the principal complement-derived anaphylatoxin *in vivo*.

All the anaphylactic peptides bind to receptors on the surfaces of mast cells and basophils and initiate the release of vasoactive amines

## The Biological Effects of Complement Activation

Table 2.1 Complement-derived anaphylactic peptides.

|  | C5a | C3a | C4a | C5a desArg |
|---|---|---|---|---|
| Amino acids | 74 | 77 | 77 | 73 |
| Molecular weight (Da) | 11 500[a] | 9080 | 8740 | 11 400 |
| Maximum concentration attainable ($\mu$M)[b] | 0.4 | 8 | 2.5 | (0.4) |
| Spasmogenic concentration (nM) | 0.5 | 10 | 1500 | 1000 |
| Permeabilization concentration (nM) | 0.0001 | 0.1 | 10 | 0.1 |
| Minimum % activation for biological effect | 0.0005 | 0.001 | 0.4 | 0.1 |

[a] C5a, unlike C3a and C4a, is a glycopeptide containing a sugar moiety of about 3 kDa molecular weight.
[b] Assuming full activation of all the available precursor molecules at the site.
Spasmogenic and permeabilization concentrations refer to the minimum concentrations required to cause these effects in experimental systems.

from intracellular granules. Released histamine and serotonin act on smooth muscle to cause contraction, and on small blood vessels to cause increased vascular permeability. Binding to receptors on neutrophils stimulates the release of lysosomal enzymes.

Only in the case of C5a have the cell surface receptors involved in anaphylaxis been characterized to any degree. Receptors for C5a (and C5a desArg) are present on neutrophils, monocytes and macrophages. They mediate the cellular response to C5a and are responsible for its removal from the circulation by internalization and degradation within the cell. The actions of the anaphylactic peptides and the important control mechanisms are illustrated in Fig. 2.1.

### 2.2.2 The chemotactic factors

Chemotaxis is the process by which cells are induced to migrate in a specific direction along a concentration gradient of a substance present in their environment. Many substances can act as chemotactic factors. Among the most important in man are those derived from complement. The ability of neutrophils to respond to a chemotactic signal is an essential part of host defence, and results in an influx of phagocytic cells into the area of infection or tissue destruction. Activation of complement at the site of inflammation results in the production of several factors which can stimulate neutrophil chemotaxis (Fig. 2.2).

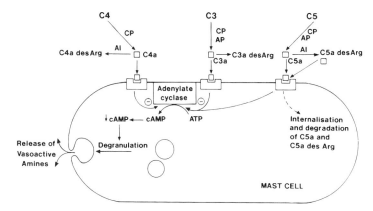

*Figure 2.1* The anaphylactic peptides.
The small peptides C3a, C4a and C5a generated during complement activation bind to specific receptors on the mast cell surface and, by downregulating adenylate cyclase, decrease intracellular cyclic AMP. The fall in cyclic AMP concentration causes the fusion of intracellular granules with the cell membranes and release of granule contents. Anaphylactic activity is regulated by the anaphylatoxin inactivator (AI) carboxypeptidase N which cleaves the C-terminal arginine from each peptide. These desArg peptides are, with the exception of C5a desArg, completely inactive. Regulation of C5a and C5a desArg activity is mediated in part by internalization and degradation of receptor-bound peptides.

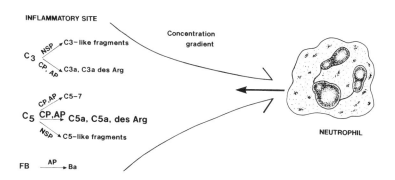

*Figure 2.2* Complement-derived chemotactic factors.
Several of the products of complement activation are chemotactic for neutrophils. Of these, C5a is the most active on a molar basis but C5a desArg is of more importance *in vivo*. All the factors diffuse away from the site of complement activation, creating a concentration gradient up which neutrophils migrate. CP, classical pathway; AP, alternative pathway; NSP, nonspecific proteases.

### 2.2.2.1 The C567 complex

The first demonstration of complement-derived chemotactic activity came from studies of the complexes formed by the terminal complement proteins. The trimolecular complex C567 induced a chemotactic response in human neutrophils, which did not occur in the presence of either of the precursors, the C56 complex or C7, alone. *In vivo*, the free C567 complex is rapidly removed from solution by binding to membranes or to fluid-phase inhibitors. It cannot therefore diffuse far from the inflammatory site and attract cells. Consequently it is unlikely to be of importance as a chemoattractant *in vivo*.

### 2.2.2.2 Chemotactic activity derived from C3 and C5

Incubation of purified C3 with the proteolytic enzyme plasmin or with any one of several other proteases yields multiple small fragments of C3 which are closely related but not identical to C3a and which are chemoattractants. It is still uncertain whether C3a itself can mediate chemotaxis but the weight of evidence seems to indicate that both C3a and C3a desArg have weak chemotactic activity. The contribution of C3-derived chemoattractants to chemotaxis *in vivo* is negligible under normal circumstances because of the far greater potency of those derived from C5.

Incubation of purified C5 with proteolytic enzymes also yields chemotactic products. The activity resides within C5a-like peptides with molecular weights of about 15 kDa. C5a itself is also a chemoattractant, the concentration range over which this activity is expressed being $0.04$–$1.7 \times 10^{-8}$ M (4–190 ng/ml). Removal of the C-terminal arginine of C5a by carboxypeptidase N reduces its chemotactic potency by a factor of 10. It has been suggested that an as yet unidentified 'helper factor' present in plasma is necessary for the expression of C5a desArg chemotactic activity. Because of its relative stability C5a desArg can diffuse long distances from the inflammatory site, recruiting inflammatory cells from a wide area. It is therefore likely to be the most important complement-derived chemoattractant *in vivo*.

### 2.2.2.3 Chemotactic activity derived from Factor B

Cleavage of the alternative-pathway component Factor B by Factor D releases a small fragment, Ba, which is chemotactic *in vitro*. Ba is a very much less potent chemotactic agent than C5a (or C5a desArg) and so is unlikely to be of much relevance to chemotaxis *in vivo*.

### 2.2.3 Other pro-inflammatory effects of C5a

As detailed above, C5a is by far the most important complement-derived anaphylactic and chemotactic factor, and therefore has a central role in the stimulation of inflammation. C5a also causes a number of other pro-inflammatory effects as a consequence of its interactions with neutrophils. The overall effect is to bring neutrophils to the site of inflammation and there to trigger release of active molecules from them. Neutrophils in the capillaries bind C5a (or C5a desArg), which causes increased cell adhesion to the capillary endothelium. The cells penetrate the vessel wall and move up the C5a concentration gradient towards the inflammatory site. Once there, again as a result of stimulation by C5a, neutrophils release reactive oxygen metabolites, eicosanoids and enzymes, all of which contribute to destruction of the initiating stimulus. This sequence of events occurring at the inflammatory focus provides an important and efficient mechanism of host defense. Activation of neutrophils by C5a at inappropriate sites or in excessive amounts causes damage to normal tissues, a pathogenic mechanism which arises many times in the later chapters of this book when the role of complement in specific diseases is discussed.

### 2.2.4 Complement-derived leucocyte mobilizing factor

A characteristic feature of any inflammatory condition is an increase in the number of circulating white cells, a leucocytosis, which makes cells available for uptake into the inflammatory site. Evidence that the factor(s) responsible for mobilizing leucocytes from their depots are complement-derived was first provided by studies of leucocytosis in complement-deficient animals and patients. Individuals deficient in C3 were incapable of mounting a leucocytosis in response to infection, implicating C3 as the source of the factor. Cleavage of purified C3 by proteolytic enzymes or by the classical-pathway C3 convertase generated a leucocyte mobilizing factor which was shown to be a low-molecular-weight (10 kDa) peptide. The purified peptide induced a biphasic leucocytosis in experimental animals, an early phase within 30 minutes of injection and a second phase peaking at about 2 hours. The peptide is derived from the α-chain of C3 but the exact portion of the chain which it constitutes is still unclear. The small (10 kDa) C3e fragment (see Fig. 2.4) has recently been implicated and receptors for this fragment have been identified on neutrophils.

## 2.2.5 The membrane attack complex as a pro-inflammatory factor

The membrane attack complex (MAC) formed by the terminal complement components C5b, C6, C7, C8 and C9 has long been considered to be a cell lysing agent. This image derives from studies of the effects of the MAC on metabolically inert target cells. Nucleated cells are, however, resistant to lysis, and formation of MACs on these cells may cause cell stimulation.

At the inflammatory site complement activation occurs and MACs are deposited on the surfaces of the invading organisms. Host cells in close proximity to the activation site will also have small amounts of MACs deposited on their surfaces (*innocent bystander* effects, see

Table 2.2 Nonlethal effects of the MAC.

| Cell | Effects | $Ca^+$ dependence |
|---|---|---|
| Neutrophil (rat) | ROM production | √ |
|  | $LTB_4$ production | √ |
| Neutrophil (human) | ROM production | √ |
|  | $LTB_4$ production | √ |
|  | Vesiculation | √ |
| Platelet (human) | Prothrombinase activation | √ |
|  | Vesiculation | √ |
|  | $TXB_2$ production | a |
| Monocyte/macrophage (human) | $PGE_2$ + $TXB_2$ production | √ |
|  | ROM production | √ |
| Glomerular epithelial cell (rat) | $PGE_2$ + $TXB_2$ production | NI |
|  | Vesiculation | NI |
|  | PL activation + $IP_3$ production | √ |
| Glomerular mesangial cell (rat) | $PGE_2$ + IL-1 production | NI |
|  | ROM production | NI |
| Oligodendrocyte (rat) | $LTB_4$ production | NI |
| Synoviocyte (human) | ROM production | √ |
|  | $PGE_2$ production | NI |
| Tumour cell lines | $LTB_4$ production | √ |
|  | Vesiculation | √ |

a Extracellular $Ca^{2+}$ not required but release of $Ca^{2+}$ from intracellular stores does occur.
*Abbreviations*: ROM, reactive oxygen metabolites; $LTB_4$, leukotriene $B_4$; $TXB_2$, thromboxane $B_2$; $PGE_2$, prostaglandin $E_2$; PL, phospholipase; IL-1, interleukin 1; NI, not investigated.
Modified from Morgan, *Biochemical Journal* **264**, 1–14 (1989), with permission.

Section 1.3.3.1). *In vitro*, nonlethal amounts of MAC have been shown to induce the production and release of reactive oxygen metabolites, eicosanoids, enzymes and other inflammatory mediators from a variety of cell types (Table 2.2). Stimulation of cells at the inflammatory site by nonlethal amounts of MAC may therefore cause further enhancement of inflammation. The interactions between the complement-derived factors involved in inflammation are summarized in Fig. 2.3.

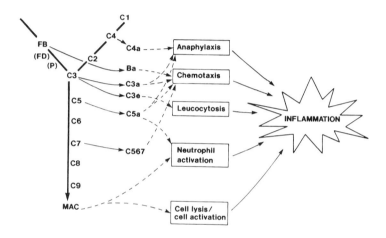

*Figure 2.3* Complement-derived inflammatory mediators.
The fragments and complexes produced during complement activation, and the pro-inflammatory effects mediated by them, are summarized. The relative importance of each mediator in the induction of inflammation *in vivo* is discussed in the text.

## 2.3 COMPLEMENT-DERIVED OPSONIC ACTIVITY

Opsonisation is the process by which foreign organisms or particles are rendered more easily ingestable by phagocytes. The process involves the coating of target particles with proteins which the phagocytic cell can then recognize and bind via specific membrane receptors. Among the most important of these coating proteins or opsonins are the bound fragments of C3 and C4 which are generated during complement activation on the particle surface. Opsonins not derived from complement, for example IgG and fibronectin, operate in a similar fashion, binding specifically (IgG) or nonspecifically (fibronectin) to the target particle and then binding via specific receptors to phagocytes. Interactions between the

## 44 The Biological Effects of Complement Activation

complement-derived and noncomplement opsonins occur and are vital for efficient phagocytosis. As an aid to understanding the structures of the opsonic fragments, the cell-bound degradation products of C3 and C4 are shown in Fig. 2.4.

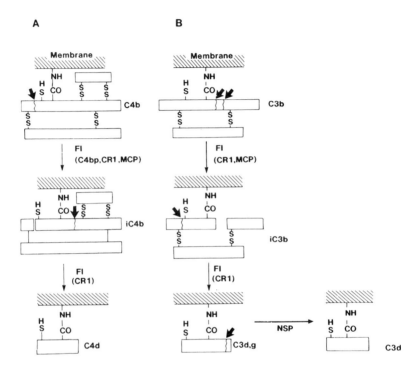

*Figure 2.4* Degradation of C3 and C4.
The membrane-bound breakdown products of C4 and C3 are illustrated as an aid to understanding the fragment specificities of the complement receptors. (A) C4 is rapidly cleaved at a single site by Factor I (FI) in the presence of appropriate cofactors to yield iC4b. A second, slow cleavage by Factor I releases a large fragment, C4c, leaving the small C4d piece attached to the membrane. (B) Cleavage of C3 by Factor I occurs initially at two sites, releasing a small fragment to yield iC3b. Further slow cleavage by Factor I releases the large fragment C3c, leaving C3d,g on the membrane. This fragment is further degraded to C3d by nonspecific proteases (NSP).

### 2.3.1 C3-derived opsonic activity

Activation of the classical or alternative pathways on a target particle causes deposition of C3b. C3b generated by the classical pathway is rapidly degraded by Factor I to iC3b, but C3b generated by the alternative pathway is protected on activator surfaces and is thus degraded much more slowly (see Sections 1.3.1 and 1.3.2). Both C3b and iC3b are opsonins; C3b is the more potent because of its higher affinity for phagocyte receptors, but iC3b is functionally at least as important because of its higher density on most target particles. C3b and iC3b not bound to receptors are further degraded by Factor I to form C3d,g and C3d, which are extremely weak opsonins.

### 2.3.2 C4-derived opsonic activity

Activation of the classical pathway on a particle surface results in the deposition of fragments of C4 as well as C3. The fragment C4b is opsonically active, binding via the same phagocyte receptors which bind C3b and iC3b but with a much lower affinity. The fragment iC4b produced by Factor I cleavage of C4b, unlike its C3-derived equivalent, has little or no opsonic activity alone. It may, however, enhance the opsonic activity of iC3b when the two molecules are present together on the target surface.

### 2.3.3 Non-complement opsonic activity

The two major noncomplement opsonins are IgG antibody and fibronectin. They are described here because of their interactions with complement-derived opsonins.

IgG opsonic activity is in most cases mediated by specific antiparticle antibodies. Some microorganisms have surface components which bind IgG nonspecifically. Once bound, IgG can interact with phagocyte receptors for the Fc portion of the molecule. Bound IgG will also activate the classical pathway, depositing fragments of C3 and C4 on the target surface and enhancing opsonisation. Three distinct types of phagocyte Fc receptors which differ in their IgG subclass specificity have so far been identified in man (FcRI, FcRII and FcRIII). Until recently it was thought that IgG was the only immunoglobulin with opsonic activity. It has now been shown that IgA can also act as an opsonin, and specific IgA receptors have been identified on phagocytes.

Fibronectin, a serum protein with a molecular weight of 440 kDa, binds nonspecifically to collagen, to certain strains of bacteria and to other microorganisms. Specific fibronectin receptors on phagocytes then bind the coated target particle. Fibronectin alone causes particle binding to the phagocyte but does not stimulate phagocytosis. When present in combination with any of the other opsonins, however, it enhances opsonic activity.

### 2.3.4 Phagocyte receptors for complement fragments

At least four types of complement fragment receptors, differing from one another in their fragment specificities, are present on the phagocyte surface. These have been named, in order of their discoveries, complement receptor types 1–4 ($CR_1$–$CR_4$). Together with the Fc receptor for IgG these cell surface molecules are essential for normal phagocytosis.

#### 2.3.4.1 Complement receptor Type 1 ($CR_1$)

The first complement receptor described, $CR_1$, was initially identified on erythrocytes and subsequently demonstrated on neutrophils and other cells (Table 2.3). $CR_1$ has the widest cellular distribution of the complement receptors. Its primary ligand is C3b but it also binds C3bi and C4b, albeit with considerably lower affinities. For effective binding to occur, interaction of ligand with receptor must be multivalent. $CR_1$ not only acts as a receptor for C3b on particles but also acts as a cofactor for Factor I in the cleavage of C3b (Section 1.3.4.1). Erythrocyte $CR_1$ has been purified and shown to be a large glycoprotein existing in four allelic forms with molecular weights of between 160 and 250 kDa. Despite these large size differences no functional difference between the allelic proteins has been detected. The $CR_1$ molecules on other cell types are antigenically indistinguishable from erythrocyte $CR_1$. Neutrophil $CR_1$ is of similar molecular weight to the erythrocyte receptor, but $CR_1$ on other cell types is about 5 kDa smaller. The number of $CR_1$ molecules on erythrocytes varies greatly between individuals but remains constant within an individual over many years.

Neutrophils and monocytes in their resting state have relatively few $CR_1$ molecules per cell (see Table 2.3) but on stimulation with chemotactic factors receptor numbers can increase 10-fold. The possible relationship between erythrocyte $CR_1$ number and the inflammatory disease systemic lupus erythematosus is discussed in Chapter 6.4.

#### 2.3.4.2 Complement receptor Type 2 ($CR_2$)

The $CR_2$ molecule is present only on B lymphocytes where it binds particles bearing the small C3d fragment of C3. It also binds C3dg, C3bi and C3b, the latter with a much reduced affinity. $CR_2$ isolated from the B lymphoblastoid Raji cell line is a 140 kDa molecule which is very susceptible to proteolytic degradation.

B lymphocytes are not phagocytically active; therefore, binding of C3 fragments to the $CR_2$ receptor cannot be involved in the clearance of foreign particles. Its role remains uncertain but it has been implicated as an enhancing factor in antibody-dependent cellular cytotoxicity (ADCC) and in lymphocyte proliferation (Chapter 2.5).

As well as binding fragments of C3, $CR_2$ also binds the Epstein–Barr virus (EBV), the causative agent of Burkitt's lymphoma and of infectious mononucleosis. Binding of EBV to $CR_2$ enables the virus to enter and infect B lymphocytes. The binding site on $CR_2$ utilized by EBV is distinct from the C3 fragment binding site.

### 2.3.4.3 Complement receptor Type 3 ($CR_3$)

The receptor $CR_3$, present only on neutrophils, macrophages and those lymphocytes involved in ADCC, has as its primary ligand iC3b. Binding of iC3b to this receptor is dependent on the presence of divalent cations. $CR_3$ is composed of an α-chain of molecular weight 183 kDa and a β-chain of 105 kDa. The β-chain of $CR_3$ is also found in two other two-chain protein molecules: LFA-1, a leucocyte surface protein involved in T-lymphocyte-mediated cell killing, and a protein known until recently as p150,95, which is present on those cells bearing $CR_3$ and is now thought to be a fourth complement receptor ($CR_4$).

The presence of $CR_3$ on phagocytes is important for normal removal of foreign particles. Individuals deficient in this receptor have impaired phagocytic function and suffer repeated bacterial infections.

### 2.3.4.4 Complement receptor Type 4 ($CR_4$)

$CR_4$, previously known as p150,95, is structurally similar to $CR_3$ (see above), is present on the same cell types and is also involved in clearance of opsonised particles. Its ligand specificity resembles that of $CR_3$ except that it does not bind zymosan in the absence of complement fragments.

## 2.4 IMMUNE COMPLEX SOLUBILIZATION AND TRANSPORT

Because antibody molecules have two antigen binding sites, interaction of antibody and antigen at high concentration *in vitro* results in the formation of a lattice which continues to grow until precipitation occurs (Fig. 2.5). *In vivo*, precipitation of these lattices or immune complexes is strongly inhibited by complement, preventing deposition of insoluble aggregates in the tissues.

Table 2.3 Complement receptors for fragments of C3.

| | Molecular weight (kDa) | Cell distribution (number per cell) | Specificity | Function |
|---|---|---|---|---|
| $CR_1$ | 190–250[a] (single chain) | Erythrocytes (500–700) Neutrophils ($4\times10^3$)[c] Monocytes/macrophages ($4\times10^3$)[c] B-lymphocytes ($2\times10^4$) Some T-lymphocytes ($1\times10^3$) Eosinophils NK cells Renal podocytes Follicular dendritic cells | C3b (C3bi)[b] | Binds C3b and acts as a cofactor for cleavage of C3b by Factor I; immune complex clearance via binding C3-containing complexes to erythrocytes/phagocytes |
| $CR_2$ | 140 (single chain) | B lymphocytes, follicular dendritic cells, NK cells | C3d,g C3d | Binds C3d,g/C3d-carrying complexes, enhances ADCC; growth stimulation; binds EBV |
| $CR_3$ | 260 (α-chain 165) (β-chain 95) | Monocyte/macrophages Neutrophils NK cells Cytotoxic T cells | iC3b | Binds iC3b-carrying complexes; important in clearance of microorganisms |
| $CR_4$ | 245 (α-chain 150) (β-chain 95)[d] | Same distribution as $CR_3$ | iC3b | |

[a] Four allelic forms of $CR_1$ exist: Type A (190 kDa, frequency 0.83), Type B (220 kDa, frequency 0.16), Type C (160 kDa, frequency 0.01) and Type D (250 kDa, frequency 0.001).
[b] Affinity of $CR_1$ for C3bi is approximately 10% of its affinity for C3b.
[c] Numbers for resting cells: increase 10–20-fold on stimulation.
[d] $CR_3$ and $CR_4$ share a common β-chain.

*Abbreviations*: NK, natural killer; ADCC, antibody-dependent cellular cytotoxicity; EBV, Epstein–Barr virus.

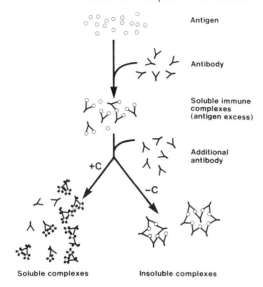

*Figure 2.5* Solubilization of immune complexes by complement.
Antigen (open circles) is bound by antibody in the circulation to form immune complexes which, in the presence of an excess of antigen, are small and soluble. Binding of more antibody in the absence of complement generates large, insoluble complexes. Complement (C, closed circles), specifically C3b, binds to the immune complexes and prevents the formation of large aggregates.

## 2.4.1 Inhibition of immune precipitation and immune complex solubilization by complement

Association of IgG or IgM antibodies with antigen in immune complexes initiates classical-pathway activation. Binding of C1 to the complex causes some inhibition of precipitation by mechanisms which are not as yet clear. C1 binding is followed by formation of the C3 convertase C4b2a and by coating of the forming immune complex with C3b. Binding of C3b to the immune complex interferes with lattice formation, thereby limiting its growth and rendering it more soluble (Fig. 2.5).

Although classical-pathway activation alone may be sufficient to prevent precipitation of nascent immune complexes, solubilization and dissipation of preformed complexes requires participation of both the classical pathway and the alternative pathway. This results in deposition of much larger amounts of C3b over the entire surface of the complex. Binding of C3b disrupts the antibody–antigen lattice by intercalating into the lattice, thereby breaking primary antigen–antibody bonds. Solubilization is maximal when about one C3b molecule is bound per antibody molecule in the complex.

## 2.4.2 Erythrocyte involvement in immune complex clearance

Many cell types, including erythrocytes, express receptors for complement fragments on their surfaces (detailed in Section 2.3.4). The receptor on erythrocytes ($CR_1$) binds C3b, particularly when this molecule is present in clusters on the surface of microorganisms or immune complexes. More than 90% of the $CR_1$ in the circulation is present on erythrocytes. Immune complexes coated with C3b thus rapidly become bound to erythrocytes, preventing precipitation regardless of the size of the complex. Binding of immune complexes to erythrocytes in blood is a dynamic process, the C3b attached to erythrocyte $CR_1$ being efficiently cleaved by Factor I ($CR_1$ acting as a cofactor in the cleavage), thereby releasing the complex. Rebinding then occurs via uncleaved C3b on the complex and the process of release and rebinding continues until all immune complex C3b is exhausted. During this process the size of the immune complex is continually reduced, rendering it more soluble. The erythrocyte membrane therefore removes immune complexes from the fluid phase and catalyses their breakdown into smaller, more soluble particles. Erythrocytes also act as a transport system for immune complexes, carrying them to the fixed macrophages of the reticuloendothelial system (primarily in the liver) where processing and breakdown take place. The mechanisms by which complexes are transferred from erythrocyte to macrophage are uncertain, but immune-complex-coated erythrocytes are neither damaged nor delayed during passage through the liver, implying that the dynamic nature of erythrocyte–complex binding is relevant, macrophages binding complexes after their release from the erythrocyte receptors (Fig. 2.6).

## 2.4.3 Clinical relevance of immune complex processing

As described above, complement and erythrocytes act together to maintain immune complexes in a soluble or cell-bound form. These factors prevent precipitation of immune complexes under normal physiological conditions *in vivo* and provide an efficient mechanism for the disposal of foreign antigen. When the system fails, however, precipitation of large, insoluble aggregates in the tissues may occur, contributing to disease pathogenesis. Failure may occur at any stage of immune complex processing. Firstly, immune complex deposition may occur when there is deficiency of a single complement

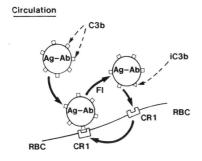

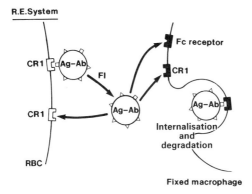

*Figure 2.6* Erythrocyte transport of immune complexes.
Immune complexes coated with C3b bind to complement receptors ($CR_1$) on the erythrocyte (RBC) surface. Once bound, C3b is susceptible to cleavage by Factor I (FI), $CR_1$ acting as a cofactor in the cleavage. As $CR_1$ does not bind cleaved C3b (iC3b), cleavage releases the immune complex from the erythrocyte. Because many molecules of C3b are present on the complex it rapidly rebinds and the cycle is repeated. Immune complex binding to erythrocytes is thus a dynamic process. In the spleen or in other reticuloendothelial sites, fixed tissue macrophages which express receptors for C3b ($CR_1$) and antibody (Fc receptor) compete with erythrocytes for binding of released immune complexes. Once bound to the macrophage, immune complexes are internalized and degraded.

component, particularly C3, C1, C4 or C2. Secondly, formation of very large amounts of immune complexes may swamp the capacity of the complement system, causing functional depletion of complement and failure to inhibit precipitation. Thirdly, abnormalities in erythrocyte $CR_1$, by diminishing the capacity of erythrocytes to process and transport complexes, may dispose to precipitation. Finally, decreased clearance of complexes by the liver may result from reduced hepatic blood flow or from defects in hepatic macrophage function. All of these malfunctions have been implicated in the pathogenesis of diseases and are discussed in detail in later chapters.

## 2.5 THE ROLE OF COMPLEMENT IN THE IMMUNE RESPONSE

Although the complement system has been studied for over a century, a role for complement in the induction of antibody response to antigen was first postulated only 15 years ago. It was initially suggested that binding of fragments of C3 to receptors on B lymphocytes was a necessary second signal for elicitation of an antibody response by bound antigen. At first this postulate was highly controversial, because of the variable results obtained using different antigens — some antigens appeared to require C3 fragment binding to elicit a B lymphocyte response, whereas others did not. Although the mechanisms are still incompletely understood it is now clear that complement, and in particular C3, has an important role in the immune response to antigen. Receptors for other complement components such as Factor H and C1q are also found on B lymphocytes and have recently been implicated in cell maturation and proliferation.

### 2.5.1 Complement and antibody responses

Human B lymphocytes express large amounts of both $CR_1$ and $CR_2$ on their surfaces, the latter receptor being present only on this cell type (Section 2.3.4). Antibodies to these receptors have been shown to stimulate B lymphocytes to proliferate and mature into immunoglobulin-secreting plasma cells, implying that receptor occupancy is a mitogenic stimulus. This implication was confirmed by the finding that insoluble aggregates of C3b (the ligand for $CR_1$) or C3d (the ligand for $CR_2$) also stimulate B lymphocyte proliferation. Evidence for the involvement of C3 fragments in the mounting of an antibody response to antigen has also been provided by utilizing the complement activating agent cobra venom factor (CVF). CVF, which is actually cobra C3b, binds factor B and properdin in serum to form a stable C3 convertase which rapidly causes complete depletion of circulating C3. Treatment of animals with CVF suppresses production of an antibody response to some but not all antigens. The antigens usually affected are those which require T cell processing — i.e. thymus-dependent antigens.

Other complement fragments also influence antibody production by B lymphocytes, at least *in vitro*. C3a inhibits antibody responses to a variety of antigens and suppresses lymphocyte proliferation, perhaps by influencing the activity of suppressor T lymphocytes. In

## The Role of Complement in the Immune Response 53

contrast, C5a enhances antibody production and lymphocyte proliferation *in vitro*. An effect of the alternative-pathway-derived fragment Ba on antibody responses *in vitro* has also recently been described.

### 2.5.2 Complement and immunological memory

Anamnesis, or immunological memory, is the ability of an animal to respond with a heightened antibody response to the second or subsequent administration of a particular antigen. It results from the generation on first exposure to antigen of a population of B memory lymphocytes primed to respond rapidly and efficiently to that antigen. A role for complement in the development of immunological memory was suggested by experiments with animals depleted of C3 using CVF. Thymectomized, C3-depleted animals failed to produce B memory cells in response to antigen whereas thymectomized animals with an intact complement system responded normally. The primary IgM response to antigen was little affected by

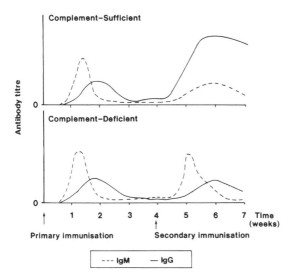

*Figure 2.7* Complement and immunological memory.
The upper trace illustrates the antibody response to injected antigen in normal animals. About 4 days after primary immunization an IgM response is detectable which is followed by a slower but longer-lasting IgG response. Boosting with the same antigen at 4 weeks produces a rapid rise in IgG titres and only a small IgM response. The primary response to injected antigen in animals depleted of C3 is unaltered, but on boosting no rapid rise in IgG titres is seen, demonstrating a failure in the development of immunological memory.

C3 depletion but on second exposure, instead of a secondary IgG response, an IgM response was once again elicited (Fig. 2.7). A similar failure to develop immunological memory has been demonstrated in animals deficient in C4, suggesting that the development of memory requires activation of complement, not merely the presence of C3.

Although the precise role of complement in the induction of B memory lymphocytes is still not certain, C3 has been shown to facilitate antigen localization and trapping in lymphoid follicles, and it has been suggested that it is this event that is essential for the development of immunological memory. Follicular dendritic cells in the lymphoid follicles of spleen and lymph nodes bind immune complexes containing C3 fragments via complement and Fc receptors on their surfaces. Antigen in these complexes is thus trapped in the lymphoid follicles where it can stimulate B lymphocyte maturation and proliferation and the development of a population of B memory lymphocytes. In the absence of C3, trapping of immune complexes in the lymphoid follicles does not occur and memory does not develop.

### 2.5.3 Role of complement in the immune response in man

A confounding problem in relating the evidence obtained from animal models to the potential role of complement in the development of an immune response in man is the finding that most individuals with deficiencies of complement components, including those deficient in C3, appear to mount a normal antibody response to antigen. It is possible that the requirement for C3 in these individuals is circumvented by the gradual acquisition of IgG antibody following repeated exposure to antigen. Normal IgG responses would then develop with time, despite the loss of C3-dependent antigen trapping capacity and B lymphocyte proliferation. Abnormal antibody responses would then only be found upon exposure to a previously unencountered antigen and it is in these early encounters that complement deficiency might be manifest as an abnormal immune response.

## 2.6 SUMMARY AND CONCLUSIONS

From the above account it is clear that complement is involved in a diverse range of biological events. Fragments and complexes produced during complement activation mobilize phagocytic cells and guide them to the site of tissue injury. There complement activation products aid neutralization of invading organisms either directly, by causing lysis, or indirectly, by stimulating phagocytes to release toxic metabolites. Phagocyte clearance of organisms and damaged tissue is enhanced by coating with complement activation products. Complement also serves vital roles in the processes of antigen clearance and immune complex solubilization and is required for optimal immune responsiveness to antigens. In Fig. 2.8 all of these functions are summarized and the important interactions between them indicated.

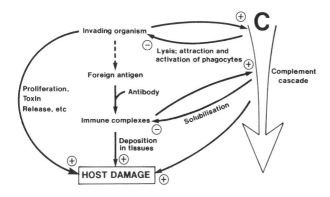

*Figure 2.8* Summary of the biological effects of complement.
Complement activation may both protect against and be responsible for injury *in vivo*. Invading organisms or immune complexes formed from antigens shed from these organisms activate complement which accelerates elimination of these agents, thus limiting host damage. However, complement activation is itself potentially damaging and if it occurs inappropriately or excessively will cause injury. +, positive effect — activation, increased damage; −, negative effect — lysis, enhanced elimination.

## 2.7 FURTHER READING

*Anaphylaxis and chemotaxis*

Bitter-Suermann, D. (1988). The anaphylatoxins. In: Rother, K. and Till, G. O. (eds), *The Complement System*. Springer, Berlin, pp. 367–395.

Hugli, T. E. (1984). Structure and function of the anaphylatoxins. *Springer Semin. Immunopathol.* **7**, 193–219.

Till, G. O. (1988). Chemotactic factors. In: Rother, K. and Till, G. O. (eds), *The Complement System*. Springer, Berlin, pp. 354–367.

*Opsonisation and complement receptors*

Fearon, D. T. (1984). Cellular receptors for fragments of the third component of complement. *Immunol. Today* **5**, 105–110.

Schreiber, R. D. (1984). The chemistry and biology of complement receptors. *Springer Semin. Immunopathol.* **7**, 221–249.

*Immune complex solubilization*

Schifferli, J. A. and Paccaud, J.-P. (1989). Complement and its receptor: a physiological transport system for circulating immune complexes. In: D'Amico, G. and Colasanti, G. (eds), *Contributions to Nephrology, Vol. 69*. Karger, Basel, pp. 1–8.

Whaley, K. (1987). Complement and immune complex diseases. In: Whaley, K. (ed.), *Complement in Health and Disease*. MTP Press, Lancaster, pp. 163–183.

*Complement and the immune response*

Klaus, G. G. B. and Humphrey, J. H. (1986). A re-evaluation of the role of C3 in the activation of B lymphocytes. *Immunol. Today* **7**, 163–165.

CHAPTER THREE
# The Genetics of Complement

## 3.1 INTRODUCTION

As in so many other fields, the advent of molecular biological techniques has revolutionized our understanding of the complement system. Within the last decade the primary sequences of the majority of the complement components and controlling proteins have been elucidated and the chromosomal locations of the genes that code for many of these proteins have been mapped. Knowledge of the primary sequence and chromosomal localization of the proteins has provided new insights into the well known polymorphic variants identified for many components, and has revealed surprising degrees of structural conservation within the system. Examination of complement component polymorphisms (and deficiencies, discussed in Chapter 4) has provided evidence of genetic linkage of many components with each other and with non-complement gene products. The important linkages are also discussed in this chapter.

## 3.2 POLYMORPHISMS OF COMPLEMENT COMPONENTS

The term *polymorphism* refers to the variations in properties of a particular protein which can be revealed by biochemical or immunological tests. Different forms of the protein are often

## 58   The Genetics of Complement

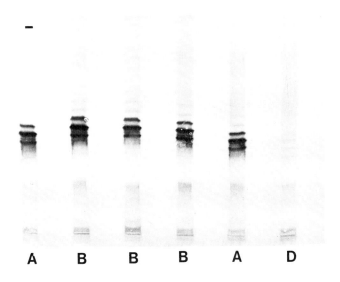

*Figure 3.1* Separation of allotypes by isoelectric focussing.
Serum samples are fractionated by isoelectric focussing in agarose gel and then transferred onto nitrocellulose paper. The transfer membrane is then probed with an appropriate antiserum, in this case anti-C6 antiserum, followed by peroxidase-labelled second antibody and developer. The C6 bands stain with antibody. The two major allotypes of C6, C6A and C6B, marked (A) and (B) respectively, are easily distinguished. The lane marked (D) contains serum from a C6-deficient individual. Cathode (marked −) at top of gel.

demonstrated by electrophoretic or antigenic heterogeneity and may occasionally exhibit marked functional differences. In this account no reference will be made to polymorphisms detectable only at the genetic level — i.e., restriction fragment length polymorphisms (RFLPs). A variety of techniques have been used to separate polymorphic variants, including agarose gel electrophoresis, isoelectric focussing and polyacrylamide gel electrophoresis, the allotypes being detected after separation by immunofixation or by Western blotting and immunoprobing using appropriate antisera. An example of the separation of allotypes by isoelectric focussing is shown in Fig. 3.1.

Polymorphic variants have been described for most of the complement proteins (the important exceptions being C1q, C8γ and C9) and are summarized in Table 3.1. The most clinically relevant and the commonest of the polymorphisms are described below.

Table 3.1 Polymorphisms of complement components.

| Component | Alleles | Frequency* | | |
|---|---|---|---|---|
| | | W | N | O |
| C4 A | 1 | 0.004 | 0.009 | — |
| | 2 | 0.080 | 0.071 | 0.106 |
| | 3 | 0.690 | 0.590 | 0.686 |
| | 4 | 0.056 | 0.036 | 0.132 |
| | QO | 0.110 | 0.273 | 0.067 |
| C4 B | 1 | 0.760 | 0.730 | 0.590 |
| | 2 | 0.100 | 0.146 | 0.167 |
| | QO | 0.136 | 0.044 | 0.158 |
| C3 | S | 0.780 | 0.950 | 0.995 |
| | F | 0.200 | 0.040 | 0.001 |
| C2 | C | 0.965 | 0.985 | 0.939 |
| | B | 0.035 | 0.015 | 0.022 |
| | A | — | — | 0.034 |
| C6 | A | 0.640 | 0.551 | 0.427 |
| | B | 0.340 | 0.403 | 0.483 |
| | B2 | — | — | 0.076 |
| C7 | 1 | 0.980 | — | 0.874 |
| | 2 | 0.010 | — | 0.081 |
| | M | 0.005 | — | 0.096 |
| C8 A | A | 0.640 | 0.700 | 0.623 |
| | B | 0.350 | 0.246 | 0.367 |
| | A1 | 0.003 | 0.054 | — |
| C8 B | A | 0.952 | — | — |
| | B | 0.044 | — | — |
| | A1 | 0.004 | — | — |
| Factor B | S | 0.710 | 0.437 | 0.801 |
| | F | 0.280 | 0.512 | 0.198 |
| Factor H | 1 | 0.691 | — | — |
| | 2 | 0.302 | — | — |
| | 3 | 0.006 | — | — |

For original references, see Rittner and Schneider (1988) in: Rother and Till (eds), *The Complement System*, Springer, pp. 89–91.
* Unfilled column spaces indicate information unavailable: W, white caucasian; O, oriental (Japanese); N, negro (American except for data on C3 and C2 which are derived from African or mixed negro population).

## 60 The Genetics of Complement

### 3.2.1 Polymorphism in C4

C4 is by far the most polymorphic of the complement proteins: at least 30 distinct polymorphic variants are known. The gene for human C4 is duplicated in the genome, one copy coding for the isotype C4A and the other for the isotype C4B which differ in sequence by only six amino acids located in short regions of the C4d fragment (40 kDa molecular weight, see Fig. 2.4). The two isotypes differ in terms of charge (C4A is more anionic) and antigenicity (C4A carries the Rodgers blood group antigen, C4B carries the Chido antigen). About 70% of the caucasian population express both isotypes, 20% express the B isotype alone, and 10% express only the A isotype. Polymorphic variants occur in both isotypes with about the same frequency, and in both involve sequence changes which are again predominantly in the C4d region. All allotypes of C4A bind preferentially via their thiolester group to amino groups on activating surfaces, activate C3 poorly and are inefficient at lysing

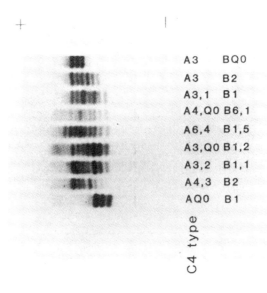

*Figure 3.2* Allotypes of C4.
Plasma has been fractionated by electrophoresis in agarose and the gel stained for C4 using anti-C4 antibodies. Complex banding patterns are seen because of the presence in plasma samples of multiple polymorphic forms of C4. From: Sim and Dodds (1987) in: Whaley, K. (ed.), *Complement in Health and Disease*, p. 100. Reproduced by permission of MTP Press Ltd., Lancaster.

sheep erythrocytes, whereas all allotypes of C4B bind preferentially to hydroxyl groups, readily activate C3 and are haemolytically efficient. Some allotypes of C4A, notably C4*A6, have extremely low lytic activity. The electrophoretic behaviour of some common allotypes of C4 is illustrated in Fig. 3.2. The patterns are often complex because each of the four loci may express a different C4 allotype.

Several of the rare allotypes of C4 have been associated with disease. The poorly lytic variant C4*A6 appears to be more common in patients with lepromatous leprosy, the C4*B2 allele appears with increased frequency in multiple sclerosis and in Alzheimer's disease, and the C4*B29 allele has been described in association with rheumatoid arthritis. The mechanisms by which the possession of specific alleles influence susceptibility to these latter diseases remain obscure, but may suggest impaired resistance to an unidentified infective agent.

### 3.2.2 Polymorphism in C3

The common allotypes of C3 are designated on the basis of their mobility in isoelectric focussing gels, as C3*F (fast-migrating) or C3*S (slow-migrating). In caucasians the allelic frequency is 0.77 for S and 0.22 for F. In persons of negro or oriental origin the F allotype is rare (less than 5% for negros, less than 1% for orientals). Within these two major categories reside a number of rare variants which exhibit small differences in mobility on focussing. The amino acid differences producing allotypic variants of C3 occur mainly in the C3d region, analogous to the site of variation in C4. No clear functional differences between the allotypes of C3 have yet been described, and there is little evidence linking specific allotypes with diseases.

### 3.2.3 Polymorphism in C2

Only one common allele for C2 has been described in man, C2*C(1), which has a frequency of over 95% in all racial groups studied. Variants are rare and no clear association between C2 structural variants and disease has been demonstrated. Studies of these rare polymorphisms have revealed close linkage in the genome between C2 and its alternative pathway homologue Factor B, variants of which are described below.

### 3.2.4 Polymorphism in Factor B

Two common allotypes of Factor B are defined by isoelectric focussing in man, slow (S) and fast (F). In caucasians and orientals the frequency of the S variant is about 80% and of the F variant about 20%, whereas in negros the F variant is the more frequent (S about 40%, F about 60%). The amino acid differences between these two major variants reside in the small Ba fragment of the molecule. Factor B*F is more haemolytically active than factor B*S *in vitro* but the functional relevance of this finding is uncertain. At least 16 rare variants have been described, resulting from amino acid substitutions in the Bb fragments of the common variants. The F1 variant, present in up to 5% of american negros, appears to be associated with juvenile onset diabetes and with renal disease.

### 3.2.5 Terminal component polymorphism

Polymorphic variants have been described for all the terminal components except C9. Variants of C5 are not present in caucasians and have been described only in individuals of Melanesian origins.

There are two common allotypes of C6, C6*A and C6*B (Fig. 3.1), their relative frequency in different racial groups varying between 0.7:0.3 and 0.4:0.6. At least 11 rare allotypes have also been described. The common variant of C7, C7*1, has a frequency of about 0.98 in caucasians and 0.85 in orientals. Several rare alleles have been described but their relative frequencies have been established only in orientals. Analysis of C6 and C7 polymorphisms in families has revealed that these proteins are closely linked in the genome, a finding confirmed by the discovery of individuals with combined deficiencies of these two proteins (see Section 4.3.4).

C8 has a very unusual three-chain heteropolymer structure, separating in denaturants into the covalently linked $\alpha$-$\gamma$ complex and the $\beta$-chain. Polymorphic variants of the $\alpha$ and $\beta$ subunits have been described but no variants of the $\gamma$-chain have yet been found. The two common variants of C8$\alpha$ (C8A variants), A and B, have relative frequencies of about 0.6:0.4 in all populations so far studied. The frequencies of variants of C8 $\beta$ (C8B variants) have been calculated only for caucasians, where the A allele has a frequency of 0.95 and the B allele of 0.05. No association of terminal component polymorphism (excluding gross deficiency) with disease has yet been found.

## 3.3 STRUCTURAL HOMOLOGIES WITHIN THE COMPLEMENT SYSTEM

All the constituent proteins of the complement pathways and many of the complement regulatory proteins have now been sequenced. This achievement has provided new insights into the way the proteins interact with one another and has also revealed that homologies exist within the system, enabling the components to be placed in groups or families whose members are functionally and structurally similar (Table 3.2). Homologies have also been demonstrated between complement proteins and noncomplement proteins with similar functional roles. The complement system therefore provides an excellent model of evolutionary conservation.

*Table 3.2* Families of homologous proteins in the complement system.

|  | Specific features | Common features |
|---|---|---|
| *Serine protease* | | |
| C1r | Highly homologous, linked | 23 kDa serine protease |
| C1s |  | domain, substrate |
| C2 | Highly homologous, linked | specificity dictated by rest |
| Factor B |  | of molecule |
| Factor I | Circulate in active form | |
| Factor D | | |
| (Trypsin) | | |
| (Chymotrypsin) | | |
| *C3-like* | | |
| C3 | Bind to membrane after | Single-chain precursor, |
| C4 | activation | multichain mature; |
| C5 |  | buried thiolester group |
| ($\alpha$-2-macroglobulin) |  | (not C5) |
| *RCA cluster* | | |
| Factor H | Soluble | Structure dominated by |
| C4bp |  | SCRs; bind C3 and/or C4; |
| $CR_1$ | Membrane-associated | cofactors in cleavage of |
| $CR_2$ |  | these molecules |
| DAF | | |
| MCP | | |
| *Terminal components* | | |
| C6 | Highly homologous, linked | Common cysteine-rich |
| C7 |  | regions |
| C8$\alpha$ | Functional and structural | Involved in cell lysis |
| C8$\beta$ | resemblance | |
| C9 | | |
| (Perforin) | | |

Non-complement proteins are bracketed.

### 3.3.1 Homologies in the enzymes of activation and control

Many of the enzymes involved in complement activation and control belong to the serine protease family. These enzymes, C1r, C1s, C2, Factor B, Factor D and Factor I, share a common catalytic region, the serine protease domain, a 27 kDa region at the carboxyl terminus of each protein. C1r and C1s are highly homologous elsewhere in the molecule, as are C2 and factor B, and it is likely that these protein pairs have arisen in evolution by gene reduplication. The genes for these proteins are discussed in detail below.

#### 3.3.1.1 C1r and C1s

Both C1r and C1s are 83 kDa proteins present free in serum and bound in intact unactivated C1 as single chain proteins with no enzymatic activity. Both are cleaved during activation at identical places to give disulphide-bonded two-chain molecules, serine esterase activity residing in the smaller of the chains (B chain, 27 kDa). The noncatalytic A chains (56 kDa) of each molecule consist of, from the N terminus, a unique series of repeating structures, a Type III cysteine-rich domain (epidermal growth factor-like) and a set of 60 amino acid short consensus repeats (SCRs) (Fig. 3.3). Both SCRs and Type III domains are found in many other complement proteins and their possible role in the interactions of components with one another is discussed later. The genes for C1r and C1s are closely linked and have been assigned to the p13 region of chromosome 12 in man.

#### 3.3.1.2 C2 and Factor B

C2 and Factor B are structurally and functionally closely related.

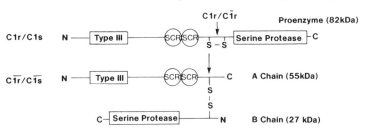

*Figure 3.3* Structure of C1r and C1s.

C1r and C1s are highly homologous molecules, each containing several conserved cysteine-rich regions, a Type III region near the N terminus and two short consensus repeats (SCRs) near the centre of the molecule. The serine protease domain is close to the C terminus. Activation of the molecule involves cleavage at a singe site; the two chains remain held together by disulphide bonds.

Both are single-chain proteins with molecular weights of about 100 kDa (about 735 amino acids) and both are serine esterases which, after activation, cleave C3 and C5. From linkage analysis of polymorphisms and deficiencies it has been known for some time that C2 and Factor B are close together in the genome. The genes have been localized in the major histocompatibility region (MHC), the region on chromosome 6 coding for the transplantation antigens. The Class III region of the MHC contains the genes for C2, Factor B and both isotypes of C4 (Fig. 3.4). Despite the close similarity between C2 and Factor B at the protein level and at the level of messenger RNA, sequencing of the genes has revealed that the C2 gene is three times the length of the Factor B gene as a result of the inclusion of additional intron sequence.

The Factor B gene comprises a 6 kilobase sequence containing 18 exons. The 5' end, encoding the Ba fragment, contains three consecutive exons each encoding a 60 amino acid short consensus repeat (SCR, see above and Section 3.2.5). The serine protease domain is at the 3' end in the area encoding the C-terminal half of the Bb fragment and is highly homologous with the other serine proteases. An additional exon in the serine protease domain and the area encoding the N-terminal half of the Bb fragment are homologous only to the C2 gene and probably confer substrate specificity on the proteins encoded by these genes.

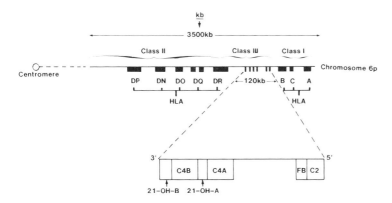

*Figure 3.4* Complement genes within the major histocompatibility locus.
The genes for complement components C4 (isotypes A and B), C2 and Factor B (FB) reside within the major histocompatibility complex (MHC), a 3500 kilobase region in the short arm of chromosome 6 which encodes the important transplantation antigens (HLA). All the complement genes have been mapped to a 120 kilobase segment in the Class III region of the MHC (expanded below) which also contains the genes for the A and B isotypes of the enzyme 21-hydroxylase (21-OH). The gene for tumour necrosis factor (TNF) is just 5' to this segment.

### 3.3.2 Homologies with C3

The complement proteins C3, C4 and C5 are highly homologous with one another. This homology is shared by the noncomplement protein α-2-macroglobulin, a protease inhibitor present in plasma. The three complement proteins are synthesized as single-chain precursor molecules which are cleaved prior to release to give the two-chain (three in the case of C4) circulating form. Each is activated by cleavage of a small fragment from the α-chain. C5, unlike the other two, does not possess an internal thiolester group and is therefore not capable of covalently binding to surfaces on activation. The amino acid sequences of the proteins reveal about 25% overall identity after alignment, homology being strongest in those areas thought to be of most functional importance. The genes encoding C3, C4 and C5 are not linked and have been localized to different chromosomes, the C3 gene to chromosome 19, the C4 genes (A and B) to the MHC on chromosome 6, and the gene for C5 on chromosome 9.

### 3.3.3 Homologies in proteins involved in control of activation

Activations of C3 and C4 are central events in the complement pathway and are therefore tightly controlled (see Section 1.3.4). The proteins involved in control at this stage in the fluid phase are Factor H and C4 binding protein (C4bp). Control on the membrane is mediated by the complement receptors $CR_1$ and $CR_2$, decay accelerating factor (DAF) and membrane cofactor protein (MCP). These six proteins, known collectively as the *regulators of complement activation (RCA) proteins*, are related structurally as well as functionally. Although very different in terms of molecular weight they are all composed mainly of 60–70 amino acid SCRs similar to those found in C1r, C1s, C2 and Factor B (Sections 3.3.1 and 3.3.5). The RCA protein chains contain between 4 and 30 SCRs. All except Factor H also contain non-SCR regions clustered at the C terminus (Fig. 3.5). The non-SCR regions are likely to dictate many of the properties which differentiate the proteins — differences in quaternary structure, ligand specificity and membrane anchoring.

The first evidence that the RCA proteins might have a common evolutionary origin came from linkage studies of polymorphic variants. These studies demonstrated that the genes encoding Factor H, C4bp and $CR_1$ are closely associated in the genome. Genetic

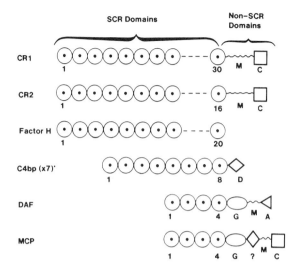

*Figure 3.5* The regulators of complement activation.
The six proteins comprising the regulators of complement activation (RCA) group are all encoded in a short segment on the long arm of chromosome 6, the RCA locus. All the proteins contain multiple short consensus repeats (SCRs) which make up the bulk of the molecule, together with a variable number of non-SCR regions clustered at the C terminus. Factor H is made up entirely of SCRs. $CR_1$, $CR_2$, complement receptors 1 and 2, respectively; C4bp, C4 binding protein; DAF, decay accelerating factor; MCP, membrane cofactor protein; M, membrane-spanning domain; C, cytoplasmic domain; D, disulphide bridge-containing domain; A, membrane anchoring domain; G, glycosylation domain; ?, domain of unknown function. C4bp consists of seven identical chains joined at a central core.

mapping has now shown that the genes for $CR_1$, $CR_2$, DAF and MCP are all located in band q32 of the long arm of chromosome 1 — the RCA cluster. The gene for Factor H, though close to this cluster on chromosome 1, has not been accurately mapped. It is therefore evident that the RCA proteins have arisen as a result of duplication and divergence of a common ancestral gene during evolution. Why this protein family, unlike the C3-related proteins and many other protein families, has remained clustered rather than spreading through the genome is unclear.

### 3.3.4 Homologies in the terminal complement proteins

The four terminal complement components C6, C7, C8 and C9 are soluble hydrophilic plasma proteins which, after cleavage of C5, assemble sequentially into a complex with C5b which is capable of inserting into membranes (see Section 1.3.3). Assembly of the membrane attack complex (MAC) occurs nonenzymatically, binding of each component into the complex exposing a binding site for the next. The complete MAC contains one molecule each of C5b, C6, C7 and C8 and up to 18 molecules of C9. C6, C7 and C9 are all single polypeptide chains, whereas C8 consists of three distinct chains two of which are disulphide-bonded ($\alpha$ and $\gamma$) and the third ($\beta$) is noncovalently associated in the complex. All four of the terminal components have now been sequenced, revealing a surprising degree of homology between them (Table 3.3).

Table 3.3 Sequence homologies between the terminal complement proteins.

| Comparison | Homology* | |
|---|---|---|
| | Overall (%) | Conservative substitutions (%) |
| C9:C8$\alpha$ | 24 | 46 |
| C9:C8$\beta$ | 26 | 47 |
| C8$\alpha$:C8$\beta$ | 33 | 53 |
| C7 (1–524):C8$\alpha$ | 28 | — |
| C7 (1–524):C8$\beta$ | 30 | — |
| C7 (1–524):C9 | 23 | — |
| C6:C7 | 29 | 52 |
| C6 (1–610):C8$\alpha$ | 26 | 52 |
| C6 (1–610):C8$\alpha$ | 22 | 48 |
| C6 (1–610):C9 | 18 | 47 |

* The first column gives the percentage of amino acids identical in the two proteins, whereas the second gives the percentage identical or substituted by a similar amino acid. For C6 and C7, comparison is made only with the N-terminal portion of the molecule, the C-terminal portions having no homologies with the other components, though considerable homology (27%) with each other.

### 3.3.4.1 Homologies between C6, C7, C8 and C9

C9, the first of the four terminal components to be sequenced, is a 538 amino acid polypeptide chain encoded by a very long (> 80 kilobases) gene on chromosome 5. Within the molecule, three-dimensional structure is dictated largely by areas rich in cysteine. Three different types of cysteine-rich domains have been identified in C9. The N-terminal 77 amino acids constitute a cysteine-rich domain which is homologous to a repeating sequence present three times in the platelet adhesive protein thrombospondin, and has been termed the Type I cysteine-rich domain. The next 40 amino acids constitute a second cysteine-rich domain (Type II) homologous to the Type A cysteine-rich sequence repeated seven times in the

LDL receptor. The third cysteine-rich domain (Type III) resides in a sequence of 35 amino acids near the carboxyl terminus of the molecule. It is homologous to cysteine-rich regions in epidermal growth factor (EGF) and to the Type B LDL receptor repeat. The terminology has been complicated by naming these domains according to their homologies (e.g. EGF-like). Here the domains are numbered according to their relative positions in C9, the first of the terminal complement proteins to be sequenced, the Type I domain being nearest the amino terminus and the Type III domain nearest the carboxyl terminus. The importance of these cysteine-rich domains in MAC assembly will be discussed later.

The unusual three-chain structure of C8 has attracted much attention. Until recently it was assumed that the disulphide-bonded α- and γ-chains were synthesized as a single-chain precursor, a finding common to most secreted proteins containing disulphide-linked subunits (including C3, C4 and C5). However, molecular cloning of C8 has demonstrated that all three subunits are encoded at different genetic loci. The genes for the α- and β-chains are located close together on the short arm of chromosome 1. Identification of the gene for the γ-chain is complicated by the absence of polymorphic variants but using specific nucleotide probes it has recently been located on chromosome 9q. The α- and β-chains of C8 are homologous to one another and to C9, whereas the γ-chain is structurally unrelated (Table 3.3). C8 γ has no homology with other complement components but is homologous with α-1-microglobulin and with protein HC, and because of these homologies a role in immunoregulation has been proposed.

The three cysteine-rich domains described in C9 (Types I, II and III) are all highly conserved in the α- and β-chains of C8 which also contain an additional Type I domain near the carboxyl terminus which is not present in C9 (Fig. 3.6).

Complement component C7 is a 821 amino acid single polypeptide chain of molecular weight 100 kDa. The gene for C7 has been localized to chromosome 12. C7 contains considerable homology with C9 and the α- and β-chains of C8 but only within the N-terminal 524 amino acids. Two Type I cysteine-rich areas are present in C7, one near the N terminus and the other in the middle of the molecule. One each of the Type II and Type III cysteine-rich areas are also present at approximately the same positions as their equivalents in the other terminal components. C7 also contains several other short cysteine-rich areas in the nonhomologous C-terminal region which are not related to the three types of segments present in C8 and C9, but are homologous with the short consensus

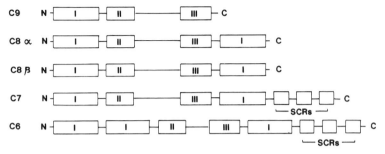

*Figure 3.6* Homologies in the terminal components.
Considerable homology exists between the terminal complement components C9, C8α, C8β, C7 and C6. Most of the homology resides within conserved cysteine-rich regions. Cysteine-rich domains Types I, II and III are present in all the terminal components, C9 containing a single copy of each, and the other components contain a single copy of Types II and III but multiple copies of the Type I domain. C6 and C7 also contain several copies of a fourth type of cysteine-rich domain, the short consensus repeat (SCR).

repeats (SCRs) found in the early components and control proteins.

C6, a single-chain glycoprotein with a molecular weight of about 110 kDa, is the first acting of the family of terminal complement components but was the last to be sequenced. As predicted from its molecular similarities and close genetic linkage, C6 is highly homologous with C7 (overall homology 34%). C6 is larger than C7, consisting of 913 amino acids. It contains Type I, Type II and Type III cysteine-rich repeats and SCRs in a similar arrangement to C7, and also contains near its N terminus an extra copy of the Type I cysteine-rich repeat present once at the N terminus of all the other terminal components. The C5b-binding domain of C6 is near the C terminus of the molecule and appears to involve the SCR domains. An SCR-mediated interaction of C7 with C5b has also been suggested to occur during MAC assembly.

### 3.3.4.2 Homologies between terminal complement proteins and perforin

Perforin is a protein molecule present in the granules of killer T cells and natural killer cells which can lyse target cells by forming MAC-like pores in the target membrane. The structural and functional similarities between the pores produced by the two effectors suggest that they induce cell lysis in similar ways and raise the possibility that perforin is structurally related to the component proteins of the MAC (see Section 1.3.3.5).

Isolated perforin is a single-chain protein with a molecular weight of 70 kDa. In the presence of calcium ions it self-polymerizes on cells to form pores in the membrane. Evidence suggestive of homologies between the terminal complement components and perforin was initially provided by studies of antibody cross-reactivities. Antibodies raised against the terminal components, particularly C9, showed variable degrees of reactivity with perforin. Cloning and sequencing of perforin has confirmed the existence of a limited degree of homology between perforin and C9, the C-terminal part of C9 being about 25% homologous with the N-terminal part of perforin. The homology includes the putative membrane binding site of C9 and the Type III cysteine-rich domain. Perforin does not contain homologues of the Types I and II cysteine-rich domains found in C9 and the other terminal complement components, the C-terminal part of the molecule having many of the features of a calcium-binding protein (Fig. 3.7). The identification of structural as well as functional similarities between perforin and the terminal complement components provides evidence for a common evolutionary origin of all these proteins. All are likely to have been derived from a common ancestral perforin-like pore forming molecule capable of nonspecifically lysing target cells, specificity in the complement membrane attack pathway arising as a result of gene reduplication and acquisition of new genetic material to produce a family of interacting proteins capable of targetted cytotoxicity (Fig. 3.8).

### 3.3.5 The building blocks of the complement proteins

From the foregoing descriptions of the structures of the components and controlling elements of the complement system it is clear that each protein is constructed from a limited number of structural domains or building blocks which are often present in multiple copies in the molecule. An important feature of all these domains is the presence of a number of highly conserved cysteine residues which form intradomain disulphide bonds, thus providing a rigid three-dimensional structure. The types of cysteine-rich domains and the complement and noncomplement proteins in which they are found are summarized in Table 3.4.

Among the early components and control proteins, the most important structural domain is the short consensus repeat (SCR). Each SCR consists of about 60–70 amino acids containing a framework of 16 highly conserved residues, including four cysteines which are disulphide-bonded to one another in a consistent way (Fig. 3.9). The SCR is a rigid triple-loop structure maintained by

## 72  The Genetics of Complement

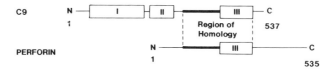

*Figure 3.7* Homology between C9 and perforin.
Comparison of the sequences of C9 and perforin reveals homology between a region near the C terminus of C9, including the Type III cysteine-rich domain, and a region close to the N terminus of perforin, which is thought to include the membrane-interactive region of perforin. Homology in these areas suggests that they may be important in the membrane binding and pore forming properties common to both these proteins.

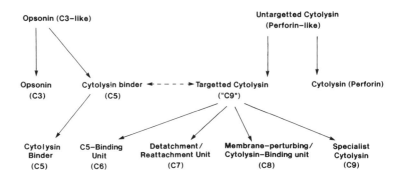

*Figure 3.8* Evolution of membrane attack pathway and perforin.
In the most primitive 'complement' system (*top*), a C3-like opsonin aids clearance of foreign particles and an unrelated cytolysin directly kills foreign cells in a rather nonspecific manner. During evolution, C5-like molecules develop out of the opsonin which can interact with a C9-like molecule derived from the original cytolysin to target cytolysin action onto the complement-activating organism (*middle*). The untargetted cytolysin persists within T-cell granules (perforin). Further evolutionary diversification of the C9-like molecule (*bottom*) produces 'specialist' molecules which bind C5 (C6), detach the forming complex from C5 and directly bind it to membrane (C7), and provide a specific binding site for the cytolysin (C8), the cytolysin itself (C9) having lost its inherent membrane binding properties.

intradomain disulphide bonds, the size of which, calculated from electron microscopic observations, is approximately 4 × 3 nm. With few exceptions each SCR is encoded by a separate exon in the gene. SCRs are present in 12 complement-related proteins and at least 3 noncomplement proteins (listed in Table 3.4). A common feature of many of the SCR-containing complement proteins (except C6, C7, C1r and C1s) is their ability to interact with C3 and/or C4 (and/or fragments of these proteins). Although it is highly likely that the

Table 3.4 Cysteine-rich domains in complement proteins.

| Type | Protein | Number | |
|---|---|---|---|
| Short consensus repeat (SCR) | C1r | 2 | |
| Approximately 60 amino acids | C1s | 2 | |
| Four conserved cysteines | C2 | 3 | |
| | Factor B | 3 | |
| | C6 | 4 | |
| | C7 | 4 | |
| | Factor H | 20 | |
| | C4bp | 56 (in 7 chains) | |
| | CR$_1$ | 30 | |
| | CR$_2$ | 16 | |
| | DAF | 4 | |
| | MCP | 4 | |
| | Factor XII | 10 | |
| | IL2 receptor | 2 | Noncomplement |
| | β2 glycoprotein | 5 | |
| Type I | C9 | 1 | |
| Approximately 60 amino acids | C8α | 2 | |
| Six conserved cysteines | C8β | 2 | |
| | C7 | 2 | |
| | C6 | 3 | |
| | Properdin | 6 | |
| | Thrombospondin | 3 | Noncomplement |
| | Circumsporozoite Protein (malaria) | 1 | |
| Type II (LDL-A) | C9 | 1 | |
| Approximately 40 amino acids | C8 | 1 | |
| Six conserved cysteines | C7 | 1 | |
| | C6 | 1 | |
| | Factor I | 2 | |
| | LDL receptor | 7 | Noncomplement |
| | Apo-E receptor | 10 | |
| Type III (LDL-B) | C9 | 1 | |
| 30–40 amino acids | C8 | 1 | |
| Four conserved cysteines | C7 | 1 | |
| | C6 | 1 | |
| | C1r | 1 | |
| | C1s | 1 | |
| | Factor I | 1 | |
| | Perforin | 1 | |
| | Urokinase | 1 | |
| | LDL receptor | 3 | Noncomplement |
| | EGF | 1 | |
| | TPA | 1 | |

## 74 The Genetics of Complement

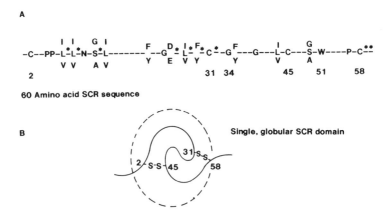

*Figure 3.9* Structure of the short consensus repeat.
The short consensus repeat (SCR) is an important component in the structure of many complement components. It consists of a stretch of approximately 60 amino acids containing a framework of highly conserved amino acids. The 22 residues shown in (A) are conserved in more than 44% of SCRs. The numbered residues, including the cysteines at positions 2, 31, 45 and 58, are conserved in over 95% of SCRs. The starred positions are occupied by charged amino acids in over 40% of SCRs. Disulphide bonds between the invariant cysteines hold the SCR in a rigid triple loop formation (B) which in some proteins can be visualized electron microscopically as a 4 nm 'bead' on the protein chain.

C3/C4 binding sites are formed by the SCRs, not all SCRs are capable of binding these components. In most of the proteins the binding site is present in the N-terminal few SCRs, the remaining SCRs in the molecule fulfilling a structural role by providing an elongated, flexible attachment of the binding site to the protein core or membrane. The recent discovery of SCRs in the C-terminal portions of the terminal complement proteins C6 and C7 has somewhat complicated the issue, as these proteins do not bind C3 or C4. A role for these domains in the binding of C6 and C7 to C5b during MAC assembly has been proposed.

The terminal components contain conserved structural domains which are distinct from the SCRs found in C3/C4 binding proteins. These domains have in common the presence of large numbers of highly conserved cysteine residues (cysteine-rich domains) and are of three main types (Types I, II and III).

The Type I cysteine-rich domain, like the SCR, consists of about 60 amino acids and contains a framework of highly conserved residues, including six cysteines. It is found in all the terminal components, C9 containing a single copy, C7, C8α and C8β containing two copies each and C6 containing three copies (Fig. 3.6). The domain is also present in the cell adhesion molecule thrombospondin (repeated three times), in the circumsporozoite protein of malaria parasites (single copy), and has recently been shown to be repeated six times in the alternative pathway protein properdin, accounting for the major part of the properdin sequence. Each domain is encoded by a separate exon in the gene and is held together by intradomain disulphide bonds. The functional role of Type I domains in properdin and the terminal components is not certain but in thrombospondin this domain is involved in binding fibrinogen and collagen, and in the malarial protein it is involved in binding of the parasite to cells. It has therefore been suggested that these domains are responsible for the protein–protein and membrane–protein interactions that occur during assembly of the alternative-pathway convertase and the MAC.

The Type II cysteine-rich domain consists of about 40 amino acids, including six highly conserved cysteine residues. It is present as a single copy near the N terminus of each of the terminal components (Fig. 3.6), and is also present twice in Factor I, seven times in the low density lipoprotein (LDL) receptor (Type A) and ten times in the apolipoprotein E receptor. In these latter molecules the domains are involved in lipoprotein binding. The efficiency of lipoproteins as inhibitors of MAC formation suggests the possibility that the Type II domains might be involved in assembly of the terminal components into the MAC.

Type III cysteine-rich domains are present as single copies in each of the terminal components (Fig. 3.6), and are also present in urokinase, epidermal growth factor, LDL receptor (Type B repeat), tissue plasminogen activator, complement components C1r and C1s and, interestingly, perforin. Each domain contains 30–40 amino acids, including four highly conserved cysteines. The presence of this domain in all the terminal components and in perforin suggests that it may have an important role in the processes of polymerization and membrane insertion that occur during formation of the MAC and of the polyperforin complex.

All three types of non-SCR cysteine-rich domains present in the terminal complement components are potentially involved in MAC assembly and this has led to the proposal of the *modular fusion hypothesis* by DiScipio. This hypothesis suggests that during MAC assembly, cysteine-rich domains (or modules) in each component bind to corresponding domains in other components sequentially and cooperatively, acting as intermolecular fasteners to maintain the proteins in their new conformations, the energy released during interdomain binding providing the driving force for unfolding and membrane insertion.

## The Genetics of Complement

Table 3.5 Known chromosomal assignments of the complement genes.

| Chromosome | Components | Comments |
|---|---|---|
| 1 | C1q | A- and B-chain genes |
| | Factor H, C4bp, MCP, $CR_1$, $CR_2$, DAF | RCA cluster, band q32 |
| | C8 α, C8 β | |
| 4 | Factor I | |
| 5 | C9 | |
| 6 | C4A, C4B, C2, Factor B | MHC Class III locus |
| 9 | C5, C8γ | |
| 11 | C1 inhibitor | |
| 12 | C1r, C1s | Closely linked |
| | C6, C7 | Closely linked |
| 19 | C3 | |
| X | Properdin | |

### 3.4 MAPPING OF COMPLEMENT GENES

From the above discussions of polymorphisms and protein families it is evident that the location of the genes coding for many of the complement proteins is known. This has been achieved in part by classical genetics, demonstrating genetic linkage between polymorphic variants of complement and previously characterized chromosomal markers. The availability of sequence data and complementary DNA (cDNA) probes derived from this sequence for most of the complement proteins has enabled genes to be localized to particular chromosomes and even to specific sites on the chromosome without the requirement for polymorphisms and defined linkages.

Assignment of complement genes to particular chromosomes has been achieved in two ways. In the first approach, *in situ* hybridization, cDNA probes tagged with radiolabel are incubated with a chromosome smear of the type used for karyotyping. The radiolabelled probe binds or *hybridizes* to its parent gene in a specific chromosome and can be localized by autoradiography. This technique allows the identification of the chromosome, and often the band on that chromosome within which the gene of interest lies. The second approach utilizes *hybridoma clones* derived from the fusion of a human cell with a rodent cell. These hybridomas lose one or more of their human chromosomes in a random fashion.

Screening of hybridomas for the gene of interest and subsequent identification of the missing chromosome(s) in those clones in which the gene is not present, allow identification of the chromosome containing that gene. The chromosomal assignments so far reported for complement components are summarized in Table 3.5.

More specific mapping of several of the complement genes has also been performed using cDNA probes. A particularly thorough and detailed example of these studies is provided by the work of Campbell and coworkers in unravelling the relationships between the complement and noncomplement genes encoded within the Class III region of the MHC on chromosome 6. For details of the techniques used and the information obtained, the interested reader is referred to the excellent reviews by this group listed at the end of this chapter.

## 3.5 FURTHER READING

Hobart, M. J. and Lachmann, P. J. (1976). Allotypes of complement components in man. *Transplant Rev.* **32**, 26–42.

Campbell, R. D., Carrol, M. C. and Porter, R. R. (1986). The molecular genetics of components of complement. *Adv. Immunol.* **38**, 203–242.

Reid, K. B. M., Bentley, D. R., Campbell, R. D., Chung, L. P., Sim, R. B., Kristensen, T. and Tack, B. F. (1986). Complement system proteins which interact with C3b or C4b. A superfamily of structurally related proteins. *Immunol. Today* **7**, 230–234.

Tschopp, J., Masson, D. and Stanley, K. K. (1986). Structural/functional similarity between proteins involved in complement- and cytotoxic T-lymphocyte-mediated cytolysis. *Nature* **322**, 831–834.

Stanley, K. K. and Luzio, J. P. (1988). A family of killer proteins. *Nature* **334**, 475–476.

Stanley, K. K. (1988). The molecular basis of complement C9 insertion and polymerisation in biological membranes. In: Podack, E. R. (ed.), *Current Topics in Microbiology and Immunology*, Vol. 140. Springer, Berlin, pp. 49–65.

Campbell, R. D., Law, S. K. A., Reid, K. B. M. and Sim, R. B. (1988). Structure, organisation and regulation of the complement genes. *Ann. Rev. Immunol.* **6**, 161–195.

Rittner, C. and Schneider, P. M. (1988). Genetics and polymorphism of complement components. In: Rother, K. and Till, G. O. (eds), *The Complement System*. Springer, Berlin, pp. 80–135.

Hourcade, D., Holers, V. M. and Atkinson, J. P. (1989). The regulators of complement activation (RCA) gene cluster. *Adv. Immunol.* **45**, 381–416.

CHAPTER FOUR
# Complement Deficiencies and Disease

## 4.1 INTRODUCTION

Congenital and/or acquired deficiencies of all of the component proteins of the classical pathway and of most of the control proteins have been described in man. Their relative frequency and clinical consequences vary enormously. Deficiencies of many of these proteins have also been discovered in experimental animals, providing essential models for complement research. This chapter is restricted to deficiencies in man, animal models being discussed only where they provide information essential to the understanding of the human condition. To set the scene, the sources of the components *in vivo* are first briefly outlined.

## 4.2 BIOSYNTHESIS OF COMPLEMENT COMPONENTS

The major source of most of the complement components and soluble control proteins is the liver. However, other tissues and cells synthesize and secrete specific proteins. Local synthesis of complement components by macrophages and other cells at sites of inflammation may be of particular importance in maintaining local concentrations of components in the tissues during activation. Methods involving measurement of protein production from cultured cells by functional or immunochemical means have now been largely superceded by the techniques of biosynthetic labelling and specific

Table 4.1 Principal sites of synthesis of complement proteins.

| Protein | Principal site | Secondary sites |
|---|---|---|
| C1q | Epithelial cells | Monocytes, macrophages |
| C1r/C1s | Epithelial cells | Macrophages |
| C4 | Liver | Monocytes, fibroblasts |
| C2 | Liver | Macrophages, monocytes |
| C3 | Liver | Macrophages, fibroblasts, etc. |
| C5 | ? Liver | ? Monocytes, ? fibroblasts |
| C6 | ? Liver | Monocytes |
| C7 | ? Liver | Monocytes |
| C8 | ? Liver | Monocytes |
| C9 | ? Liver | Monocytes |
| Factor B | Liver | Monocytes/macrophages |
| Properdin | Monocytes | ? |
| Factor D | Monocytes | Adipose tissue, lung |
| C1inh | Liver | ? |
| Factor I | Liver | Monocytes |
| Factor H | Monocytes | ? |

mRNA analysis. Table 4.1 lists the principal sources of the complement proteins in man.

The complement proteins are broadly divisible into three groups on biosynthetic grounds: those proteins made and secreted as a single chain (e.g. C6, C7); those made as a single chain but processed intracellularly and secreted as a disulphide-bonded multichain molecule (e.g. C3, C4); and those which are composed of multiple, separately synthesized chains (products of distinct genes) assembled prior to secretion (e.g. C1q, C8).

C2 is synthesized as a single chain in the liver and also in macrophages and monocytes. Factor B, which is closely linked to C2 within the major histocompatibility complex (MHC), is made by the same cells in concert with C2. The terminal components, C6, C7, and C9, are all synthesized and secreted as single-chain proteins. The site of synthesis of the terminal components is still uncertain but is likely to be primarily the liver. Biosynthesis of all the terminal complement components by monocytes has recently been reported.

C3, C4 and C5 are all made as single chain precursors which undergo post-translational modification prior to secretion to yield the disulphide-bonded multichain circulating molecule. Intracellular processing of all three molecules is similar, each is synthesized in a precursor form which is cleaved by intracellular enzymes (Fig. 4.1). Examination of serum C3 allotypes prior to and following liver transplantation has demonstrated clearly that this organ is the

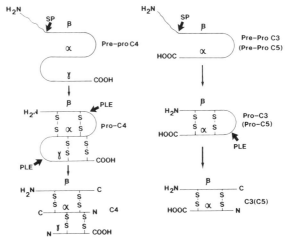

*Figure 4.1* Biosynthesis of C3, C4 and C5.
C3, C4 and C5 are all biosynthesized as single-chain molecules. Within the cell the signal peptide is removed and the molecules become folded, disuphide bonded and finally cleaved by intracellular enzymes to form the multichain mature protein. Glycosylation and other modifications also occur prior to release from the cell. SP, signal peptidase; PLE, plasmin-like enzyme.

primary source of C3 in man; however, many other cell types, including fibroblasts and macrophages, can produce C3 (Table 4.1). The liver is also the primary source of plasma C4. Extrahepatic C4 synthesis occurs in monocytes and macrophages. The major site of synthesis of plasma C5 in man remains controversial. Evidence for hepatic and monocyte C5 biosynthesis has been reported.

Biosynthesis of C1q is complex. The complete molecule is assembled within the cell from 18 component chains — six copies of each of three distinct protein chains, the products of separate genes. The source of plasma C1q is still uncertain but the weight of evidence appears to favour epithelium, particularly intestinal and urogenital epithelium. C8 is also assembled intracellularly from the products of three separate genes. As for the other terminal components, monocyte synthesis of C8 has recently been reported but the source of plasma C8 has not yet been identified conclusively.

### 4.3 COMPLEMENT DEFICIENCIES IN MAN

Most complement component deficiencies in man are inherited but some clinically important examples of acquired deficiency also exist. Unless otherwise stated all the deficiencies discussed in this section are hereditary. Hereditary complement deficiencies may result from markedly diminished or absent synthesis of a component or from the synthesis of an abnormal, functionally inactive molecule. Heterozygous deficiencies usually result in plasma levels of the component of about one-half the normal value, and do not predispose to any disease. Deficiency of C1 inhibitor (C1inh) is the exception to this rule, heterozygous deficiency resulting in plasma levels well below 50% and in clinical disease (hereditary angioedema; see below). Although heterozygous deficiencies do not, as a rule, cause disease they may serve as genetic markers for specific diseases. For example, heterozygous C2 deficiency, though not causally related, is present with increased frequency in patients with systemic lupus erythematosus (SLE), juvenile rheumatoid arthritis and glomerulonephritis.

Homozygous deficiencies have been recognized for all the complement components and control proteins with the exceptions of Factor B, C4 binding protein (C4bp) and Factor D. All the deficiencies are relatively rare, and the incidence varies greatly between different ethnic groups. In the caucasian population C2 deficiency is the commonest, whereas in the Japanese by far the commonest is deficiency of C9 — a very rare finding in other racial groups. Homozygous deficiencies are often, though not always, associated with disease. The known deficiencies, their relative frequencies and disease associations are summarized in Table 4.2. Deficiencies of components belonging to the same pathway within the complement system give rise to similar clinical problems (Fig. 4.2). The major features and clinical consequences of the important deficiencies are detailed in the following sections.

## 4.3.1 Deficiencies of classical-pathway components

Deficiency of any of the three subcomponents of C1 will block classical pathway activation. C1q deficiency is relatively common. It is caused either by a failure to synthesize C1q (about 60% of cases) or by the synthesis of a functionally inactive (though immunochemically detectable) molecule (40%). In the latter case the diagnosis can be made only by assays of function, as immunochemical assays detect normal or increased amounts of C1q.

Deficiencies of C1r or C1s are less common and result from a failure to synthesize these subcomponents. Combined deficiency of both subcomponents has been described, a consequence of their close genetic linkage. Lack of a functioning C1 molecule gives rise to

Table 4.2 Complement deficiencies in man.

| Component | Number of cases[a] | Associated diseases |
|---|---|---|
| C1q | 13 | Pyogenic infections, SLE, GN |
| C1r/C1s | 9 | |
| C4 | 13 | |
| C2 | 77 | About 50% healthy, remainder SLE, GN, infections |
| C3 | 14 | Severe immune deficiency, SLE, GN |
| C5 | 13 | Meningococcal meningitis, gonococcal sepsis, SLE |
| C6 | 33 | Meningococcal meningitis, SLE (rare) |
| C7 | 22 | |
| C8 | 31[b] | |
| C9 | 4[c] | Healthy, meningococcal meningitis (see below) |
| Factor I | 6 | Severe pyogenic infections |
| Factor H | 2 | Haemolytic uraemic syndrome |
| Properdin | 4 | Meningococcal meningitis, pneumonia |

[a] Up to 1984, data in part from Ross and Densen, *Medicine* **63**, 243–273 (1984).
[b] About 25% C8 A deficiency, 75% C8 B deficiency.
[c] Non-Japanese patients only. In Japan, C9 deficiency is extremely common (about 1:1000) and is apparently asymptomatic.

a spectrum of autoimmune disorders which reflect the inability to process immune complexes in the absence of a functioning classical pathway — systemic lupus erythematosus (SLE), discoid lupus erythematosus (DLE), SLE-like disease, vasculitis, glomerulonephritis, arthritis, etc. Recurrent infections, particularly of the skin and gut, are also common.

Absence of C2 also blocks activation of the classical pathway. However, the block in this situation is less complete, some C1-initiated complement activity persisting as a consequence of a recently described 'C2 bypass pathway' in which C1 directly cleaves C3. C2 deficiency is the commonest homozygous complement deficiency in caucasians, occurring in about 1 in 30 000 individuals. It results from a failure to synthesize C2, no C2-like protein being detected in the plasma. Deficiency of C2 is often associated with decreased levels (but never absence) of Factor B, reflecting their close genetic linkage. The clinical picture of C2 deficiency closely resembles that described above for C1, albeit usually with less

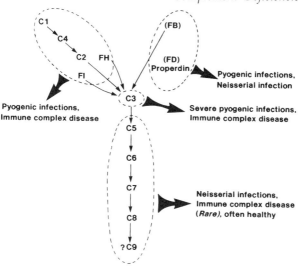

*Figure 4.2* Complement deficiencies and disease.
Deficiencies of components of the same pathway cause similar clinical problems. Classical-pathway component deficiencies commonly cause pyogenic infections and immune complex diseases, as does deficiency of C3, although infections tend to be more severe with this latter deficiency. Deficiencies of Factors H and I cause secondary depletion of C3 and thus symptoms similar to those of C3 deficiency. Alternative pathway component deficiencies are rare. Properdin deficiency specifically predisposes to neisserial infection. Terminal component deficiencies also commonly present with neisserial infection.

severe symptoms. Immune complex disease and increased susceptibility to infection predominate, but vasculitis, purpuric rashes and polymyositis are more common in the absence of C2. About one-quarter of individuals with C2 deficiency are apparently healthy.

Complete C4 deficiency requires the inheritance of null alelles at both C4 loci (C4A and C4B) and is thus rare. Individuals with complete deficiency have the typical clinical picture of a classical pathway block. Deficiency of C4A, the isotype which binds preferentially to amino groups and has low haemolytic activity, causes immune complex disease of severity comparable to that associated with complete absence of C4. Deficiency of C4B, the isotype which binds hydroxyl groups on surfaces and has high haemolytic activity, is not associated with severe disease but may be associated with vasculitis in some individuals. The reasons for these differences in the clinical consequences of C4 isotype deficiency are not clear, but are thought to relate to defective handling of immune complexes rich in amino groups in the absence of C4A.

### 4.3.2 Deficiencies of alternative pathway components

It is interesting to note that of the three proteins specific to the alternative pathway, Factor B, Factor D and properdin, complete deficiency has been described only for properdin. Partial (heterozygous) deficiencies of Factor B and Factor D have been reported, in the latter case associated with recurrent infections. Although no firm evidence exists, these findings imply that the possession of an intact alternative pathway is essential for fetal or neonatal survival.

Unlike all the other complement deficiencies, which are autosomally inherited, properdin deficiency is transmitted as an X-linked recessive trait. Thus all deficient individuals so far reported are male. Until recently properdin deficiency was considered to be very rare, but a recent spate of case reports, particularly from Scandinavia and Holland, suggests that it may not be uncommon. Males with properdin deficiency typically present with meningococcal infections which can be fulminant and life-threatening. These individuals have an intact classical pathway and on second encounter with the organism can mount a normal response. Recurrent infection is therefore not a feature of this deficiency, and screening of male relatives of the index case and immunization of deficient individuals will remove the risk. There is no evidence of increased susceptibility to immune complex disease or to infections with organisms other than the meningococcus.

### 4.3.3 Deficiency of C3

C3 is the cornerstone of the complement system. It is an essential component of both the classical and alternative activation pathways and is necessary for initiation of the membrane attack pathway. Despite this central role, several individuals have been described who completely lack C3. For reasons which are not clear, C3 deficiency, unlike other autosomally inherited complement deficiencies, is not equally common in males and females: over 80% of the reported cases of C3 deficiency have been in females.

The clinical picture of C3 deficiency resembles that seen in deficiencies of classical pathway components. Recurrent infections are the predominant feature, and immune complex diseases, particularly glomerulonephritis, are common. The severity, frequency and diversity of infections occurring in C3 deficiency may initially suggest a diagnosis of agammaglobulinaemia.

### 4.3.4 Deficiencies of the terminal components

Absence of C5 not only blocks membrane attack complex (MAC) formation but also removes the source of the most important complement-derived anaphylactic and chemotactic factor, C5a. C5-deficient individuals are therefore susceptible to repeated infections with a wide variety of organisms. Inability to form a functional MAC renders them more susceptible to neisserial infections (meningococcal and gonococcal), lysis by the MAC being a major mechanism for neutralizing these organisms (Chapter 5). Susceptibility to these infections is thus a feature common to all the terminal component deficiencies.

Lack of C6 is the second most common complement deficiency in caucasians. Nearly 50 individuals with homozygous deficiency have so far been described and its incidence in the caucasian population is about 1 in 60 000. Most cases of C6 deficiency present with recurrent meningococcal infections. A minority present with immune complex diseases, particularly SLE, and at least 25% of the reported cases are healthy.

Deficiency of C7 produces a clinical picture identical to that seen in the absence of C6. Meningococcal infections again predominate, with a few individuals having immune complex diseases. Two unrelated cases of combined deficiency of C6 and C7 have been reported, reflecting the close genetic linkage between these components. Interestingly, despite extremely low levels of functionally and immunochemically detectable C6 and C7, neither of these individuals had any symptoms which could be attributed directly to their deficiencies.

C8 deficiency may result from a defect in synthesis of either the α–γ complex (C8A deficiency) or the β-chain (C8B deficiency). In either case, the absence of a functional C8 molecule results in a clinical picture similar to that seen with deficiencies of C6 or C7. Meningococcal infection again predominates, occasional individuals presenting with immune complex disease. Rarely, C8 deficiency is associated with chronic pyogenic infections or with xeroderma pigmentosa.

Deficiency of C9 is rare in caucasians, only four cases having been reported thus far. Of these, two presented with meningococcal disease and the others were healthy. In the Japanese population, however, a very different situation is seen. C9 deficiency is by far the commonest homozygous complement deficiency in Japan, with an incidence approaching 1 per 1000. This incidence would make this deficiency one of the commonest genetic abnormalities in the

Japanese population, 1 in 16 individuals carrying a copy of the defective gene. No disease association has been found with C9 deficiency in this population. It has yet to be ascertained whether C9 deficiency in caucasians, which is rare and appears to be associated with disease, differs qualitatively or quantitatively from deficiency in the Japanese, which is common and not disease related. Recent reports indicate that deficiencies of other terminal complement components are also more common in Japan than elsewhere and, like C9 deficiency in this population, are not associated with disease. Further investigation is required to discover the reasons for these anomalous findings.

The mechanisms by which deficiencies of terminal complement components predispose to immune complex disease remain obscure. There is no evidence that these proteins are involved in immune complex solubilization, but it has been suggested that an intact complement system, including the ability to make MACs, is required for the efficient elimination of viruses and other microorganisms (Chapter 5). Deficiency of a terminal component may slow clearance of these organisms, allowing them to persist long enough to invoke an abnormal immune response and hence disease.

A common feature of deficiencies of all the terminal components is an increased susceptibility to meningococcal disease. Specific features of meningococcal disease which increase the likelihood of an underlying terminal component deficiency are summarized in Table 4.3. As noted earlier, properdin deficiency also predisposes to meningococcal disease. The features suggestive of underlying properdin deficiency are also listed in Table 4.3. The presence of any of these features in a patient with meningococcal disease should alert suspicion and initiate investigations of complement function.

### 4.3.5 Deficiencies of the controlling proteins

The complement system is a cascade pathway with a considerable potential for amplification of the initiating stimulus. It therefore requires tight regulation to prevent overactivation and consequent deleterious effects. Regulation is provided by a number of fluid-phase and membrane-associated proteins (see Section 1.3.4), deficiency of which can lead to loss of control of the whole system or of a particular reaction within the system. Regulation may also be disturbed by the presence of abnormal factors which counter the effects of the control proteins. Disturbances in control arising in both of these ways are described in this section.

Table 4.3 Features of meningococcal disease suggestive of complement deficiency.

*Features suggestive of terminal component deficiency*
  Age of onset ⩾ 10 years
  Mild, recurrent infections
  Family history*
  Infection with unusual serogroups (X,Y,Z, W135)
  Meningococcal septicaemia

*Features suggestive of properdin deficiency*
  Male
  Age of onset ⩾ 10 years
  Family history* (restricted to males)
  Severe, fulminant, nonrecurrent infection
  Infection with unusual serogroups
  Mengingococcal septicaemia

* Family history is of particular significance if the interval between cases exceeds 30 days.

### 4.3.5.1 Deficiency of C1 inhibitor

In the classical pathway, control is exerted at the stage of C1 activation by the plasma protein C1 inhibitor (C1inh) which dissociates the multimolecular C1 complex. C1inh inhibits several other serum proteases, including plasmin, kallikrein and Factors XIa and XIIIa of the coagulation system, but whereas alternative serum inhibitors of these other proteases exist, C1inh is the sole serum inhibitor of C1. Deficiency of C1inh thus results in loss of control of classical pathway activation, which manifests itself clinically as recurrent attacks of acute oedema. C1inh deficiency may be inherited or acquired, the resultant disease, angioedema, is similar in either case. In some individuals inherited C1inh deficiency is also associated with immune complex disease, presumably a result of consumption of classical pathway components leading to secondary deficiency. Unlike the other complement deficiency-associated diseases which only present in the homozygote, hereditary angi-oedema (HAE) is inherited as an autosomal dominant trait. The incidence is about 1 in 150 000 of the population and it is equally common in men and women. No cases of homozygous deficiency of C1inh have been described. In most cases of HAE (about 85%) the plasma contains low levels of normal C1inh (usually less than 30% of the normal mean). In the remaining 15% the plasma contains normal or elevated levels of a functionally defective C1inh molecule. At least two distinct types of defective C1inh have so far been identified. In individuals with decreased amounts of normal C1inh, the levels found are always much lower than the 50% of the mean predicted in heterozygous deficiencies. This is probably the result of the way that C1inh is catabolized *in vivo*. Most of the catabolism occurs as a consequence of C1inh binding to and inactivating C1 and will therefore continue at much the same rate (since just as much activated C1 is formed) even when C1inh levels are low. The combination of a *normal* rate of catabolism with a decreased rate of synthesis will reduce plasma levels of C1inh well below 50%.

The typical clinical picture in HAE consists of recurrent episodes of painless swelling in localized areas of the skin (commonly on the limbs, face and genitalia), often accompanied by an erythematous rash. In some cases oedema may also involve the gut wall and the respiratory tract. Attacks are self-limiting, usually lasting for 48–72 hours. Swelling in the subcutaneous layers of the skin is usually precipitated by minor, often unnoticed, trauma. Gut involvement, by causing temporary obstruction, causes abdominal cramps, vomiting and diarrhoea. Laryngeal involvement is a medical emergency, increasing stridor rapidly leading to airway obstruction and death if untreated. The mechanisms bringing about episodic swelling in circumscribed areas remain uncertain. It has been suggested that low-level activation of complement and plasmin at an extravascular site, perhaps following trauma, causes local exhaustion of C1inh and loss of control. Following an attack, C2 and C4 levels are decreased systemically, indicating that intense local activation has occurred. A cleavage product of C2, C2 kinin, has been implicated as the causative factor for oedema, although others have proposed that the mediator responsible is the noncomplement kinin, bradykinin.

Treatment of acute attacks of HAE involves infusion of plasma or, preferably, partly purified C1inh. Long-term therapy involves either reducing C1 activation using plasmin inhibitors such as *e*-aminocaproic acid and tranexamic acid, or increasing the plasma level of C1inh using enhancers of synthesis — anabolic steroids such as oxymethalone and danazol.

Acquired C1inh deficiency occurs in patients with benign or malignant B-cell lymphoproliferative disorders. It is a rare disorder and is thought to be the result of an anti-idiotypic immune response to the monoclonal immunoglobulin on the B-cell surface. Interaction of the anti-idiotypic antibody with B-cell immunoglobulin causes large-scale chronic activation of C1 and hence consumption of C1inh. Lack of C1inh results in angioedema, the clinical features closely resembling those of the hereditary disease. Where the diagnosis is in doubt HAE can be distinguished from acquired

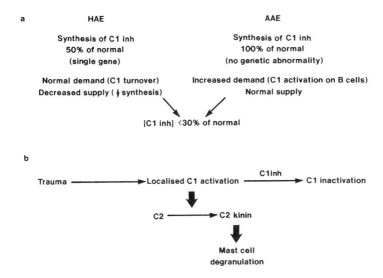

*Figure 4.3* Hereditary and acquired angioedema.
(*a*) Both hereditary angioedema (HAE) and acquired angioedema (AAE) are caused by a decrease in the plasma C1 inhibitor (C1inh) concentration. In HAE this results from a heterozygous deficiency of C1inh, reducing the biosynthetic rate to the point where normal demand outstrips supply. In AAE, synthesis of C1inh is normal, but abnormal C1 activation increases demand to the point where again supply is outstripped. Symptoms are rare until C1inh concentration is less than 30% of normal.
(*b*) At a site of trauma, C1inh is utilized to inhibit C1 and other proteases locally. If plasma levels are low the local concentration of C1inh may fall rapidly to zero. Uncontrolled activation of C1 then occurs, releasing active kinins.

angioedema by measurement of plasma C1q concentration, which is markedly decreased in the acquired disease. The main features of the two types of angioedema are summarized in Fig. 4.3.

### 4.3.5.2 Deficiencies of Factor I and Factor H

Factor I is a fluid-phase inhibitor of the C3 and C5 convertases of both the alternative and classical pathways. Homozygous deficiency of Factor I causes loss of control of the positive-feedback amplification loop of the alternative pathway, resulting in consumption of C3 and Factor B and to a lesser extent of the terminal components (Fig. 4.4). These individuals are thus rendered secondarily deficient in many components, particularly C3 and Factor B, and the clinical manifestations are the result of these secondary deficiencies. The clinical picture in Factor I deficiency is very variable between individuals, from severe, repeated infections with diverse organisms in some, to normal health in others. Occasional associations with meningococcal infections and immune complex disease have been noted. The reasons for this wide spectrum of clinical consequences are not known.

Factor H is an essential cofactor for the efficient cleavage and inactivation of C3b by Factor I in the alternative pathway positive feedback loop (Fig. 4.4). Deficiency of Factor H therefore also causes overactivation of the pathway and consumption of components, particularly C3 and Factor B, resulting in the same clinical consequences as Factor I deficiency. For reasons which are not clear, infection is not a prominent feature in the few cases of Factor H deficiency so far described, most patients presenting with immune complex disease.

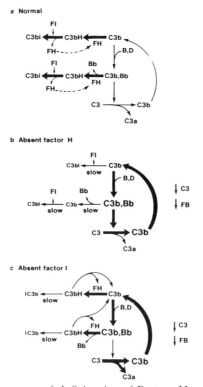

*Figure 4.4* Consequences of deficiencies of Factors H and I.

Factors H and I (FH, FI) are vital for the control of the alternative-pathway positive feedback loop. In the normal situation (*a*), Factor H binds to C3b, displacing bound Bb and rendering C3b susceptible to cleavage by Factor I. In the absence of Factor H (*b*), dissociation of the C3b,Bb complex and cleavage of C3b by Factor I are both greatly slowed, resulting in uncontrolled activation of the feedback loop and depletion of C3 and Factor B. In the absence of Factor I (*c*), C3b decays only slowly and the available Factor H is swamped with C3b. Uncontrolled activation thus ensues, consuming C3 and Factor B.

### 4.3.5.3 Deficiencies of complement receptors

The complement receptors $CR_1$, $CR_2$ and $CR_3$, present predominantly on circulating cells, bind fragments of C3 (and C4) and act as cofactors in the further breakdown of these fragments, as well as having an essential role in phagocytosis and immune complex clearance (see Section 2.3.4).

Several patients have been described who are completely deficient in $CR_3$. These individuals present in childhood with a characteristic immune deficiency syndrome consisting of repeated infections, particularly of the skin and mucous membranes, which heal leaving paper-thin scars. The symptoms closely resemble those seen in patients with neutrophil dysfunction and it appears that the immune deficiency is a consequence of an inability of the $CR_3$-deficient neutrophils to mount a respiratory burst in response to a phagocytic stimulus. Neutrophils and other cells in these individuals also lack the related molecules LFA-1 (a cell adhesion molecule) and $CR_4$, the underlying defect being an inability to synthesize the β-chain common to all three of these molecules (Section 2.3.4.3). The contributions of these other deficits to the immune deficiency have not been assessed.

Although complete deficiency of $CR_1$ has not been described, the receptor quantity on red cells is determined genetically. Individuals may have high (HH), intermediate (HL) or low (LL) numbers of $CR_1$ per erythrocyte. An inverse relationship between the number of $CR_1$ per erythrocyte and the incidence of systemic lupus erythematosus (SLE) has been demonstrated, stimulating the proposal that an inherited relative deficiency of $CR_1$ in SLE is of pathogenic importance. However, present evidence indicates that low $CR_1$ levels in SLE are a consequence rather than a cause of the disease.

### 4.3.5.4 Deficiencies of membrane-bound control proteins

Several membrane proteins are involved in the control of complement activation, including decay accelerating factor (DAF), membrane cofactor protein (MCP) and the complement receptors $CR_1$ and $CR_2$ (see Section 1.3.4). Because these proteins are involved in the control of membrane-bound convertases, deficiencies do not result in large-scale complement activation and secondary deficiency of components. Distinct clinical syndromes are, however, associated with these deficiencies.

Perhaps the best understood of these syndromes is *paroxysmal nocturnal haemoglobinuria* (PNH) — a rare, acquired disorder characterized by episodes of complement-mediated haemolysis. PNH is caused by a somatic mutation of a pluripotential haematopoietic stem cell in the bone marrow resulting in an expanding clone of abnormal cells. Because the mutation arises in a pluripotential stem cell, all elements of the circulating cell population — erythrocytes, leucocytes and platelets — are involved. The abnormal cells have a membrane defect rendering them unduly sensitive to complement lysis, resulting in episodes of intravascular haemolysis and thrombosis. Haemolytic episodes occur during periods of stress and are particularly frequent at night (as the name implies), perhaps reflecting small increases in the *tick-over* activation of the alternative pathway and thus increased complement activation on the cells at these times. In an individual with PNH the erythrocytes can be classified according to their degree of complement sensitivity, into PNH I ('normal'), PNH II (intermediate sensitivity) and PNH III (marked sensitivity). The proportions of the three phenotypes vary between individuals, those with the highest proportion of Type III cells having the most severe haemolysis.

The basic defect in PNH cells is a deficiency of the membrane proteins which normally regulate complement activation. The cells are either completely or partly deficient in decay accelerating factor (DAF), an important regulator of classical- and alternative-pathway C3 convertases, and have also recently been shown to lack two membrane proteins involved in control of lysis by the MAC (Section 1.3.4.3). The combination of these deficiencies results in increased susceptibility to lysis by complement. All three of these control proteins are attached to the membrane by means of an unusual inositol-containing lipid anchor (Fig. 4.5). Other erythrocyte membrane proteins utilizing this type of anchor, including acetylcholinesterase and the cell adhesion molecule LFA-3, are also deficient on PNH cells, implying that the underlying biochemical anomaly is an inability to make these anchors efficiently.

Recently, several individuals have been described who, because of a primary biosynthetic defect, completely lack DAF but possess normal amounts of the other inhibitors. These individuals have no haemolytic problems, implying that lack of the MAC inhibitors is of more significance in the pathogenesis of PNH. Although it has been assumed that the three types of PNH cells are qualitatively different, present evidence suggests that the differences are only quantitative, Type I cells, though deficient, retaining sufficient residual inhibitor to resist lysis and Type III cells having insufficient.

PNH may be diagnosed by demonstrating the susceptibility of the erythrocytes to complement lysis under hypotonic conditions (sucrose lysis test) or in acidified serum (acidified lysis test). Apart from transfusion to ameliorate the anaemia no effective treatment

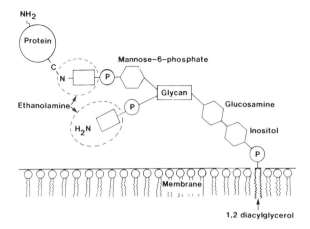

*Figure 4.5* Structure of the glycosyl phosphotidylinositol anchor.
Many proteins, including several complement control proteins, are known to be attached to the membrane through a glycosyl phosphatidylinositol (GPI) anchor. The anchor has the structure shown above. Diacylglycerol in the membrane attaches the multicomponent chain which binds via an ethanolamine residue to the C-terminal region of the protein. The structure of the glycan component is variable. The enzyme phosphatidylinositol-specific phospholipase C (PIPLC) cleaves the anchor between the diacylglycerol and inositol residues, freeing proteins attached in this way. Modified from Low, *Biochem. J.* **244**, 1–13 (1987), with permission.

for PNH exists. Thromboembolic episodes, a consequence of the defective platelets, are the most frequent serious complication of PNH and may be fatal. In a proportion of people the benign clonal expansion may, after many years, undergo malignant transformation to produce an acute leukaemia.

*Hereditary erythroblastic multinuclearity with a positive acidified serum test* (HEMPAS) is a very rare disorder which is in many ways similar to PNH. The erythrocytes are abnormally sensitive to complement lysis, resulting in haemolytic anaemia. The membrane defect in HEMPAS has not been identified, but the erythrocytes are positive (i.e. lysed) in the acidified lysis test but not in the sucrose lysis test, implying increased susceptibility to lysis by the MAC.

### 4.3.5.5 Nephritic factors causing complement deficiency

The control proteins described above act to limit the lifetimes of the complement convertases. Deficiency of these proteins extends the active life of the convertases, causing overactivation and secondary complement deficiency. Another way that the lifetime of the convertase can be increased is by binding a stabilizing factor which inhibits its decay. Properdin is the only naturally occuring stabilizing factor in plasma, it binds to and inhibits decay of the alternative-pathway C3 convertase. Abnormal stabilizing factors, known as nephritic factors, occur in association with disease. Nephritic factors are autoantibodies which bind to and inhibit decay of the C3 convertases. The first described, and most studied, of these factors is the C3 nephritic factor (C3NeF), also known as nephritic factor of the amplification loop (NFa). C3NeF is an IgG autoantibody which recognizes and binds to Factor B in the C3b,Bb complex, rendering it resistant to spontaneous or Factor-H-mediated decay. It is about 200 times more efficient at protecting the C3b,Bb complex against Factor-H-mediated decay than is the natural stabilizer properdin, and increases the half-life of the complex in the fluid phase up to 20-fold. The molecular events that occur during stabilization are not known. Overactivation of the alternative-pathway feedback loop, occurring mainly in the fluid phase, causes consumption of C3 and Factor B but the levels of early and terminal components are little changed. C3NeF is often found in patients with membranoproliferative glomerulonephritis (MPGN) Type II and with partial lipodystrophy, and occasionally in patients with MPGN Type I (Section 6.3).

C4 nephritic factor (C4NeF), also known as nephritic factor of the classical pathway (NFc), is an autoantibody which reacts with an epitope expressed on C4 within the C4b2a complex. It has been found in patients with poststreptococcal glomerulonephritis and SLE. Its role in pathogenesis is uncertain.

Nephritic factor of the terminal pathway (NFt) is an autoantibody which binds to and stabilizes the C3b,Bb,P complex. By increasing the lifetime of the alternative-pathway C3 and C5 convertases it causes consumption of C3, C5 and the terminal components. NFt has been found in patients with MPGN Types I and III. Activation of complement by this factor occurs only slowly *in vitro* and, although potentially nephritogenic, its relevance to disease pathogenesis is uncertain. The sites of action of the nephritic factors are illustrated in Fig. 4.6.

## 4.4 COMPLEMENT DEFICIENCIES AND DISEASE

From the foregoing account it should be clear that complement deficiencies, although uncommon, are associated with a relatively well-defined group of diseases. Deficiencies of complement components should be considered in patients with autoimmune diseases such as SLE and membranoproliferative glomerulonephritis, and in

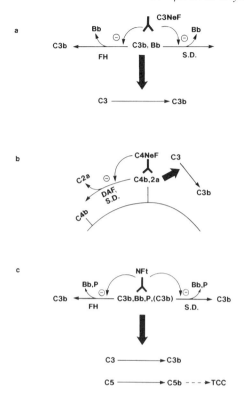

*Figure 4.6* Sites of action of nephritic factors.

(*a*) C3 nephritic factor (C3NeF) binds to Factor B in the C3b,Bb complex, inhibiting spontaneous (S.D.) or Factor H (FH)-mediated decay of the complex and thus enhancing C3 activation. (*b*) C4 nephritic factor (C4NeF) binds C4 in the C4b,2a complex, inhibiting spontaneous or decay accelerating factor (DAF)-mediated decay of the complex and thus enhancing C3 activation. (*c*) Nephritic factor of the terminal pathway (NFt) binds to and stabilizes the alternative-pathway C3 and C5 convertases, enhancing activation of these components and initiating terminal pathway activation.

patients with a history of repeated infection, particularly where the causative organism is the meningococcus. Suspicion should be heightened if either or both of these disease groups are present in several members of a family. Diagnosis requires a careful evaluation of the complement system, the methods for which are described in Section 12.2.

## 4.5 FURTHER READING

*Biosynthesis*

Colten, H. R. (1976). Biosynthesis of complement. *Adv. Immunol.* **22**, 67–118.
Colten, H. R. (1986). Genetics and synthesis of components of the complement system. In: Ross, G. D. (ed.), *Immunobiology of the Complement System.* Academic Press, London, pp. 163–182.
Whaley, K. (1980). Biosynthesis of the complement components and the regulatory proteins of the alternative pathway by human blood peripheral monocytes. *J. Exp. Med.* **151**, 501–509.

*Hereditary angioedaema*

Davis III, A. E. (1988). C1 inhibitor and hereditary angioneurotic edema. *Ann. Rev. Immunol.* **6**, 595–628.
Agostoni, A. (1989). Inherited C1 inhibitor deficiency. *Complement Inflamm.* **6**, 112–118.

*Paroxysmal nocturnal haemoglobinuria*

Schreiber, R. D. (1983). Paroxysmal nocturnal haemoglobinuria revisited. *N. Engl. J. Med.* **309**, 723–725.
Halperin, J. A. and Nicholson-Weller, A. (1989). Paroxysmal nocturnal haemoglobinuria: a complement-mediated disease. *Complement Inflamm.* **6**, 65–72.

*Other deficiencies*

Fries, L. F., O'Shea, J. J. and Frank, M. M. (1986). Inherited deficiencies of complement and complement-related proteins. *Clin. Immunol. Immunopathol.* **40**, 37–49.
Haeney, M. R., Thompson, R. A., Faulkner, J., Mackintosh, P. and Ball, A. P. (1980). Recurrent bacterial meningitis in patients with genetic defects of terminal complement components. *Clin. Exp. Immunol.* **40**, 16–24.
Ross, S. C. and Densen, P. (1984). Complement deficiency states and infection: epidemiology, pathogenesis and consequences of Neisserial and other infections in an immune deficiency. *Medicine* **63**, 243–273.

# CHAPTER FIVE
# Complement and Infectious Diseases

## 5.1 INTRODUCTION

Neutralization and removal of invading organisms constitute the major biological role of the complement system in man. As described in Chapter 1, the discovery of the complement system more than 100 years ago emanated from studies of the capacity of fresh serum to lyse certain strains of bacteria. Later it was demonstrated that serum complement, though capable of lysing directly only a few strains of bacteria, enhances phagocytosis of many other strains — the process of opsonisation (Section 2.3). This chapter describes the mechanisms by which the complement system, either alone or in concert with other facets of the immune system, eliminates bacteria, viruses, fungi and other invading organisms. The importance of these mechanisms is graphically illustrated in patients with deficiencies of complement components, many of whom suffer from severe, repeated infections with many different organisms (Chapter 4).

## 5.2 COMPLEMENT AND VIRAL INFECTIONS

### 5.2.1 Virus structure and replication

Viruses are stucturally and functionally unique among infecting organisms. The basic structure consists of a single strand of DNA or

RNA together with some associated proteins (the core) surrounded by a protein coat (the capsid). Most viruses also have an outer coating of lipid and carbohydrate (the envelope) which is not a product of the virus but is acquired from the host cell in which the virus matures. Host membrane proteins are excluded from the envelope but virus-derived proteins are present (Fig. 5.1). These viral envelope proteins are also often expressed on the surface of the host cell.

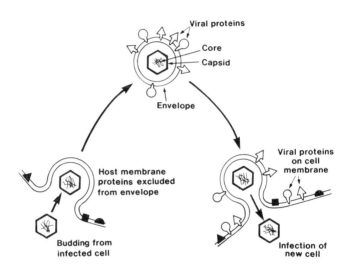

*Figure 5.1* The structure and life-cycle of a virus.
The structures and life-cycles of viruses are extremely diverse and this figure seeks only to describe some common features. Virus particles bud from infected cells taking with them an envelope derived from the host cell membrane. The infective virus consists of an envelope (derived from the host cell but expressing only viral proteins), an inner capsid and a central core containing the viral nucleic acid. Upon encountering a new target cell the virus envelope fuses with the cell membrane, releasing viral proteins to the membrane and the virus particle to the cytoplasm.

Viruses cannot proliferate independently, but once within the host cell they utilize the reproductive machinery of the cell to synthesize viral proteins and to copy viral nucleic acid. Infection of a cell by a virus initially requires tight binding of the virus to the cell membrane, usually via a specific receptor. This receptor requirement limits the range of cells which a specific virus can infect. Proliferation of the virus within the cell and subsequent release of new viral particles can damage or destroy the cell directly.

## 5.2.2 Complement activation by viruses

Viruses cause many diseases in man, and elaborate host defences against infection have evolved. Complement has an important role to play in the immune response to virus infection. On first exposure to a virus no specific antiviral antibodies are present in the host and defence resides with naturally occurring activities. Independent of complement, viruses or virus-infected cells (which express viral antigens and abnormal nonviral antigens) may be recognized and neutralized directly by macrophages, natural killer (NK) cells or neutrophils. Complement may be activated on viruses or infected cells via the classical pathway by pre-existing antibodies reactive against other viruses or against antigens which cross-react with the viral surface. Alternatively, complement may be activated directly on some viruses and virus-infected cells either via the alternative pathway or by antibody-independent activation of the classical pathway. The viruses known to activate complement independently of antibody either on the viral particle itself or on infected cells are listed in Table 5.1. These mechanisms may be of great importance in limiting the infectivity of viruses *in vivo*.

Sialic acid content is a major factor in determining whether a surface supports alternative-pathway activation, thus, as the viral envelope is host-cell-derived, viral sialic acid content and hence the complement activating capacity of a particular virus is dependent on the host cell. Some viruses can modify the host cell membrane. For example, the mumps virus carries the sialic-acid-removing enzyme neuraminidase in its envelope and can therefore decrease the sialic acid content of the envelope and of the host cell membrane, rendering the virus and host cell more susceptible to complement activation. The infectivity of this virus is consequently inversely proportional to its neuraminidase content.

The viral proteins present on the envelope and on the host cell membrane are immunogenic and thus induce an immune response in the host. On second infection with the same virus the host is primed with specific antiviral T- and B-cell clones which efficiently neutralize the virus via cellular and humoral mechanisms. Antiviral antibodies produced by the B cells not only activate the classical pathway of complement but also greatly enhance alternative pathway activation on viruses and infected cells. On infected cells antiviral antibody also has an essential but as yet undefined role in cell lysis following alternative pathway activation.

Very recently it has been demonstrated that cells infected with the *Vaccinia* virus synthesize and secrete a virally encoded protein which

Table 5.1 Activation of complement by viruses and infected cells.

| Pathway | | |
|---|---|---|
| Antibody-independent alternative | *Viruses:* | Sindbis<br>Epstein–Barr |
| | *Infected cells:* | Measles<br>Epstein–Barr<br>Sindbis |
| Antibody-independent classical | *Viruses:* | Sindbis<br>Newcastle Disease<br>Epstein–Barr<br>Retroviruses (including HIV) |
| | *Infected cells:* | — |
| Antibody-dependent alternative | *Viruses:* | Influenza |
| | *Infected cells:* | — |
| Antibody-dependent classical | *Viruses:* | Measles<br>*Herpes simplex*<br>Parainfluenza<br>Influenza<br>Vaccinia |
| | *Infected cells:* | Many |

is homologous with the complement control protein, C4 binding protein, and inhibits complement activation. Secretion of complement inhibitory proteins may occur in other viral infections and this process may represent an important strategy for viral survival *in vivo*.

### 5.2.3 Neutralization of viruses by complement

Antibody–complement-mediated neutralization of virus may be achieved by several mechanisms. Firstly, antibody — alone or in combination with complement — may cause viral aggregation. This mechanism operates even at low antibody titres and efficiently reduces the number of infective particles but does not completely neutralize infectivity. Deposition of C3 on the virus surface markedly enhances aggregation.

Secondly, deposition of antibody and complement on the viral surface will mask viral antigens, preventing interaction with receptors on susceptible cells. Deposition of C3 is required for efficient masking and neutralization. This is probably the major mechanism of neutralization for most viruses *in vivo*, but only works efficiently following classical pathway activation.

Thirdly, MAC formation on viral particles can cause lysis by disrupting the envelope and capsid and releasing the core proteins and nucleic acid. Although most enveloped viruses can be lysed *in vitro* by complement, large amounts of antibody and complement are required. Thus *in vivo*, MAC-mediated lysis appears to be the primary neutralizing mechanism only for retroviruses, and only primate complement causes lysis of retroviruses.

The final mechanism of virus neutralization involves interaction of antibody and complement on the viral surface with Fc and complement receptors on phagocytic cells. Binding of coated virus particles is followed by ingestion and destruction within the cell. The various mechanisms of viral neutralization are summarized in Fig. 5.2.

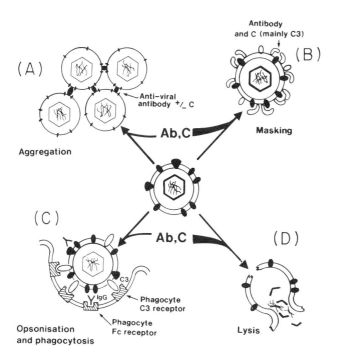

*Figure 5.2* Neutralization of viruses by complement.
(A) Viral aggregation, induced by antibody plus or minus complement, reduces the number of infective particles. (B) Masking of viral antigens by C3b prevents interaction of virus with receptors on the target cell. (C) C3b and antibody on viral surface bind to phagocyte receptors, inducing internalization and degradation of virus. (D). Formation of the membrane attack complex on susceptible viruses causes lysis.

### 5.2.4 Removal of virus-infected cells

Virus-infected cells are removed either by interaction with specific T cells or by complement-mediated lysis. It is clear that specific antiviral antibody is essential for complement lysis of infected cells, yet it is equally clear that lysis requires activation of the alternative pathway of complement. Alternative pathway activation may be triggered by virus-induced changes in the cell membrane or may be secondary to limited activation of the classical pathway, but the classical pathway alone is not able to cause cell lysis. Antibody is primarily involved at the lytic stage rather than at the activation stage but the mechanism by which it contributes to this process is unknown. Using purified components to establish the protein requirements, it has been shown that properdin is also essential for lysis of virus-infected cells. Like antibody, properdin appears to be required at the lytic stage rather than during alternative pathway activation. Again the underlying mechanism is unknown (Fig. 5.3).

### 5.2.5 Biological relevance of complement in viral infections

Although complement is undoubtedly capable of neutralizing many types of virus *in vitro*, the relevance of complement-mediated

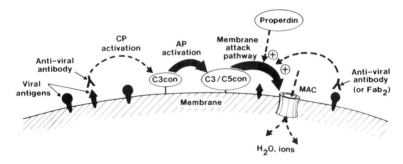

*Figure 5.3* Complement lysis of virus-infected cells.
Complement is initially activated on the surface of the infected cell either by nonspecific C3b deposition or by limited classical pathway (CP) activation mediated by antiviral antibodies. The surface of the cell is modified so that it favours amplification via the alternative pathway (AP), many AP C3/C5 convertases thus being rapidly formed. Cleavage of C5 initiates the membrane attack pathway. Both antiviral antibody (intact or Fab$_2$ fragment) and properdin play essential permissive roles at the stage of membrane attack, although the mechanisms by which they act are unknown. Formation of sufficient membrane attack complexes (MACs) on the cell surface will cause lysis.

neutralization to defence against viral infection *in vivo* is not proven. Mice depleted of C3 and C5 by treatment with cobra venom factor (CVF) and mice congenitally deficient in C5 develop more severe infections with influenza virus than normal mice, but in man individuals with deficiencies of complement components do not appear to be at increased risk of viral infections. It is likely that host defence against viral infections *in vivo* involves multiple distinct mechanisms, including NK cells, cytotoxic T lymphocytes and complement, failure of any one mechanism being adequately compensated for by the others.

The contribution of complement activation to pathogenesis in viral infections must also be considered. Acute, severe viral infections are often accompanied by marked systemic complement activation and immune complex formation. A striking example of acute symptoms following viral infection is seen in *dengue haemorrhagic fever*, where infection in the presence of pre-existing antibody results in severe haemolysis and shock. Although not proven, complement activation products have been implicated in the causation of these symptoms.

## 5.3 COMPLEMENT AND BACTERIAL INFECTIONS

### 5.3.1 Bacterial structure and complement activation

Host defence against pathogenic bacteria is determined mainly by the ability of the host immune system to damage the bacterial cell wall. The structure of the cell wall thus dictates whether and how complement can effect neutralization of the organism. On the basis of their staining reaction with Gram's reagent, bacteria can be broadly divided into two groups: Gram-positive organisms which bind the dye avidly, and Gram-negative organisms which do not. Within each group the structure of the cell wall is broadly similar, Gram-negative organisms possessing an outer lipid bilayer not present in Gram-positive bacteria (Fig. 5.4). Because of these differences the two groups of organisms also differ in their reactivity with complement.

A major component of the cell wall in Gram-negative bacteria is lipopolysaccharide (LPS), which consists of a lipid moiety (lipid A) and a polysaccharide component. Lipid A binds and activates C1 and is therefore a potent activator of the classical pathway. C1 binding to LPS is inhibited by the polysaccharide component which can itself activate the alternative pathway. As a result, strains of bacteria in which the LPS contains little polysaccharide ('rough strains') activate primarily via the classical pathway, whereas those that contain abundant polysaccharide ('smooth strains') activate via the alternative pathway.

The cell walls of Gram-positive bacteria do not contain LPS but are composed mainly of peptidoglycan (a disaccharide polymer) and teichoic acid (a glycolipid). The peptidoglycan layer can be extremely thick — up to 150 nm in some strains. These bacteria do not activate the classical pathway directly but do activate the alternative pathway in the absence of antibody. In general, Gram-positive bacteria, because of their thick peptidoglycan layer, are resistant to the bacterolytic action of complement and the major role of complement in defence against these organisms is to enhance phagocytosis.

Some bacterial strains possess a further barrier outside the cell wall, the capsule, which is composed mainly of polysaccharide.

### 5.3.2 Bacterial killing by complement

The cell walls of both Gram-positive and Gram-negative bacteria activate complement in the absence of antibody, the former via the alternative pathway, the latter via both pathways. Fragments of C3 will thus be deposited on the surface of the organism, opsonising it for phagocytosis (see Section 2.3). On some Gram-positive organisms, C3 binding and interaction of bound C3b with phagocyte receptors are inhibited by specific membrane proteins, for example the M protein of *Staphylococcus pyogenes*.

The presence of a capsule also protects bacteria from killing by complement and most pathogenic strains are encapsulated. The capsule is a porous structure, allowing plasma proteins to reach the cell wall. It is thus not an absolute barrier to complement activation on the cell, but impairs phagocytosis because complement fragments deposited beneath the capsule are not accessible to complement receptors on phagocytes. Complement fragments on the capsule are accessible to complement receptors but activation on the capsule is restricted by the presence of large amounts of sialic acid. Effective complement activation on and opsonisation of encapsulated strains occurs only in the presence of specific anticapsular antibody which enhances alternative-pathway activation by the capsule and overcomes the protective effect of capsular sialic acid. In some strains anticapsular antibody also activates the classical pathway, further enhancing C3 deposition and opsonisation.

Opsonised bacteria bind to phagocyte complement (and immunoglobulin) receptors and are phagocytosed. An involvement of complement in the process of intracellular killing has been proposed. Killing of some strains within the phagocyte appears to require the presence of antibody and complement outside the cell, although it is difficult to envisage the mechanism by which these extracellular factors contribute. Some Gram-negative strains are killed more efficiently in the cell if MACs have been formed on the bacterium prior to phagocytosis. It is likely that the MAC weakens the bacterial membrane, enhancing the effectiveness of cellular bactericidal agents.

### 5.3.3 Complement lysis of Gram-negative bacteria

Most Gram-positive organisms are, because of the very thick peptidoglycan layer in their cell walls, resistant to complement lysis. In contrast, many Gram-negative organisms, particularly *Neisseria* and *Haemophilus* species, are susceptible to lysis. The cell wall of Gram-negative bacteria consist of several layers (Fig. 5.4). Lysis of

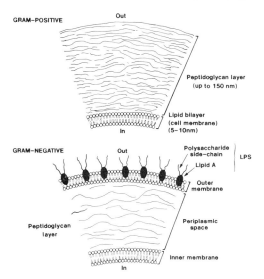

*Figure 5.4* Cell walls of Gram-positive and Gram-negative bacteria.
In Gram-positive organisms (*top*) the cell wall is composed of a very thick peptidoglycan layer which protects the single lipid bilayer. The cell wall in Gram-negative organisms (*bottom*) consists of an outer lipid bilayer in which are embedded lipopolysaccharide molecules, a central periplasmic space which contains peptidoglycan, and an inner lipid bilayer.

these organisms by the MAC is therefore more complex than lysis of an erythrocyte, which possesses only a single bilayer. It is clear that lysis requires disruption of the inner, cytoplasmic membrane but during complement attack MACs are formed on the outer membrane. The mechanisms by which this event leads to disruption of the inner membrane and lysis remain contentious. Disruption of the outer membrane releases enzymes from the periplasmic space and allows lysozyme to enter the space, destroying the peptidoglycan layer. However, this is not in itself sufficient to cause lysis. It is possible that MACs may form on the inner membrane after the outer membrane and peptidoglycan layers have been stripped away. The rapidity of lysis of sensitive strains make this sequence of events unlikely. It has been suggested that the lethal event may occur at regions of the bacterial cell wall where the outer and inner membranes are fused with no intervening periplasmic space — the Bayer adhesion zones. MAC formation at these sites may simultaneously disrupt both membranes and cause lysis (Fig. 5.5). An alternative possibility, supported by some elegant experimental evidence, is that a small fragment of the terminal component C9 is released from MACs on the outer membrane into the periplasmic space, migrates to the inner membrane and disrupts it (Fig. 5.5). A final puzzling feature of bacterial lysis by the MAC is that it appears in many strains to be energy-dependent. Blockage of cellular metabolism renders sensitive organisms resistant to killing — the converse of the situation in eukaryotic cells where cellular energy stores are utilized in protection mechanisms.

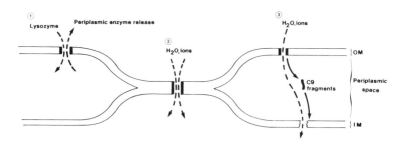

*Figure 5.5* Mechanisms of lysis of Gram-negative bacteria.
(1) Formation of membrane attack complex (MAC) on outer membrane. This event in itself does not disrupt the inner bilayer and thus cannot cause cell lysis. (2) Formation of MAC on Bayer adhesion zone. MAC formation in these regions, where inner and outer membranes are closely apposed, may cause lysis directly. (3) Release of lytic peptides. It is suggested that formation of the MAC on the outer membrane is accompanied by release of lytic fragments of C9 which migrate to and disrupt the inner membrane. OM, outer membrane; IM, inner membrane.

Resistant strains of bacteria avoid lysis by the MAC primarily by preventing its insertion into the outer membrane: just as many MACs are deposited on these organisms, but they are located on the long strands of smooth LPS which thus act as a physical barrier preventing MAC insertion into the membrane. Removal of LPS renders these strains susceptible to lysis. Some resistant strains do not have LPS molecules with long side chains to prevent MAC deposition. The mechanism of resistance in these bacteria is not known.

### 5.3.4 Biological relevance of complement in bacterial infections

The importance of complement in defence against bacterial infections is not in doubt. Patients deficient in complement components are more susceptible to a variety of infections and in complement sufficient individuals most pathogenic bacteria are complement-resistant. The role of complement in defence is dictated by the surface characteristics of the infecting organism (whether it is Gram-positive or Gram-negative, whether it posesses a capsule, whether it has specific inhibitory proteins in its cell wall), and by the presence or absence of specific antibacterial antibodies in the host. The primary complement-dependent killing mechanism for most organisms is opsonisation followed by phagocytosis, but some strains, particularly of *Neisseria*, are cleared primarily by MAC-induced lysis. Infections with these latter organisms are thus frequent in individuals with terminal component deficiencies. The molecular events occurring during complement lysis of bacteria remain an intriguing mystery.

### 5.4 COMPLEMENT AND OTHER PATHOGENIC ORGANISMS

The role of complement in the immune response to infections with agents other than viruses and bacteria has been studied relatively little. Most of these other organisms are parasitic and are present in the host for long periods. They have therefore in many cases developed elaborate strategies to evade destruction by the host immune system.

### 5.4.1 Complement and fungal infections

Complement activation by fungi has not been investigated to any great extent. Isolated fungal polysaccharides and other surface components from *Candida albicans, Cryptococcus neoformans* and *Aspergillus* spp. have been shown to activate complement via the alternative pathway in the absence of antibody, and limited data suggest that the intact organisms also activate complement in this manner. Guinea pigs treated with cobra venom factor (CVF) to deplete C3 and C5 were rendered highly susceptible to infection with *Candida albicans* and *Cryptococcus neoformans*, whereas C4-deficient animals were not more susceptible than normal animals, implying that alternative-pathway activation is important in the control of fungal infection *in vivo*. The relevance of complement activation to the elimination of fungal infection in man is not certain, although a few individuals with complement deficiencies (particularly of terminal components) appear to have an increased susceptibility to these organisms.

### 5.4.2 Complement and parasitic infections

Parasitic infections differ from most bacterial and viral infections in that they are usually very long-lasting, the organism persisting in the host for many years and establishing an equilibrium in which host damage is restricted to ensure survival of host and parasite. In order to survive in the host parasites have evolved a variety of strategies for avoiding destruction by complement, and in some cases have even turned complement to their advantage, utilizing the system to enhance their infectivity. A complicating factor in the study of parasite interactions with complement is the multiple morphological forms of the organism which appear during its life cycle. Complement may be activated well by some forms of the organism but not at all by others. In general, the more mature forms of the organism activate complement less well.

The interaction of *schistosomes*, the organisms responsible for bilharzia (schistosomiasis), with complement has received most attention. The primary form in the newly infected host, the schistosomulum, is at first susceptible to lysis by serum complement *in vitro*, although no evidence for lysis *in vivo* has been found, probably because its location in the skin protects it from serum. Once in the host the schistosomulum rapidly develops resistance to complement killing. Resistance does not involve a reduction in complement activation by the organism but represents diminished susceptibility to opsonisation and lysis, the mechanisms of which are unclear.

The flagellate *Leishmania*, responsible for Kala-azar (leishmaniasis), is an obligatory intracellular parasite of macrophages. The morphological form of the organism present in the newly infected host is sensitive to complement but only during its logarithmic growth phase. The mature, intracellular form of the organism is sensitive to alternative-pathway activation and killing but only in the presence of antibody.

*Plasmodium*, the protozoan responsible for malaria, is also an obligatory intracellular parasite, residing in erythrocytes. Although complement activation directly by the organism has not been demonstrated, infected erythrocytes activate via the alternative and, in the presence of antibody, classical pathways. Lysis does not ensue but deposition of early components stimulates phagocytosis, thus clearing infected cells. The closely related organism *Babesia*, an erythrocyte parasite of rodents and cattle which only rarely infects humans, utilizes complement to facilitate its entry into cells. Deposition of C3b on the surface of the organism allows its attachment to C3b receptors on the erythrocyte and subsequent entry into the cell. Inhibition of complement activation markedly

Table 5.2 Parasite sensitivity to complement.

| Organism | Stage | Sensitivity | Pathway |
|---|---|---|---|
| Schistosome | Cercariae | +++ | ADCP |
| | Schistosomulum (d1) | ++ | AIAP |
| | Schistosomulum (d3) | +/− | |
| | Adult schistosome (d7) | − | |
| *Leishmania* | Promastigote | +/−* | ADCP |
| | Amastigote | ++* | ADAP |
| *Trypanosoma* | Epimastigote | ++ | AIAP |
| | Trypomastigote | +/− | ADCP |
| *Echinococcus* | Protoscolex | ++ | AIAP |
| | Adult | ++ | AIAP |
| *Entamoeba* | Trophozoite (noninvasive) | +++ | AIAP |
| | Trophozoite (invasive) | +/− | |

* Promastigotes utilize complement to gain entry into cells, and amastigotes, though complement-sensitive, are intracellular and thus protected.

d1–d7, days after infection; ADCP, antibody-dependent classical pathway; AIAP, antibody-independent alternative pathway; ADAP, antibody-dependent alternative pathway.

decreases parasitaemia following innoculation of rats with *Babesia*.

The sensitivities of several important parasites to the action of complement at various stages in their life cycle are summarized in Table 5.2.

### 5.4.3 Complement, parasitic infection and immune complex disease

Parasites reside within the host for long periods and continuously release foreign antigen into the host circulation. Immune complexes will therefore be formed in the host circulation, activate complement and cause pathology. The commonest manifestation of immune complex formation is renal disease. Renal impairment may be acute and transient, as occurs commonly during the early stages of malarial infection, or may be chronic resulting eventually in renal failure. Immune complex deposition may also be responsible for many of the other pathological features of parasitic infections, including the vasculitis and carditis of Chagas' disease and the ocular damage of oncocerciasis. As in other immune complex diseases, complement has both negative and positive roles. Complement helps maintain immune complexes in solution, preventing their deposition in the tissues, and also solubilizes precipitated complexes. Activation of complement by immune complexes in the tissues will, however, exacerbate inflammation and tissue damage. As a result of chronic activation, many individuals with parasitic infections are complement-depleted and may be susceptible to other infections.

## 5.5 COMPLEMENT AND THE CONTROL OF PATHOGENS

Complement, either alone or in combination with other components of the immune system, plays an important role in controlling and eliminating invasion by a wide variety of infective organisms ranging in complexity from viruses to multicellular parasites. Complement activation on the organism may occur spontaneously or only in the presence of specific antibody. Deposition of complement on the surface of the organism is not always sufficient to initiate elimination, many pathogens escaping undamaged because of their diverse resistance strategies. The increased incidence of infective episodes among individuals with inherited complement deficiencies provides evidence of the role of complement and also enables identification of the organisms for which complement is an important neutralizing factor, and of the parts of the system involved in elimination.

## 5.6 FURTHER READING

*Complement and viral infections*

Hirsch, R. L. (1982). The complement system — its importance in the host response to viral infection. *Microbiol. Rev.* **46**, 71–85.

Cooper, N. R. and Nemerow, G. R. (1986). Complement-dependent mechanisms of virus neutralisation. In: Ross, G. D. (ed.) *Immunobiology of the Complement System*. Academic Press, Orlando, pp. 139–162.

*Complement and bacterial infections*

Taylor, P. W. (1983). Bactericidal and bacteriolytic activity of serum against Gram-negative bacteria. *Microbiol. Rev.* **47**, 46–83.

Clas, F. and Loos, M. (1987). Complement and bacteria. In: Whaley, K. (ed.), *Complement in Health and Disease*. MTP Press, Lancaster, pp. 201–231.

*Others*

Cohen, S. and Warren, K. S. (1982). *Immunology of Parasitic Infections*, 2nd edn. Blackwell, Oxford.

Vignali, D. A. A., Bickle, Q. D. and Taylor, M. G. (1989). Immunity to Schistosoma mansoni *in vivo*: contradiction or clarification? *Immunol. Today* **12**, 410–416.

Cooper, N. R. and Nemerow, G. R. (1989). Complement and infectious agents: a tale of disguise and deception. *Complement Inflamm.* **6**, 249–258.

CHAPTER SIX
# Complement and Renal Disease

## 6.1 INTRODUCTION

An involvement of the immune system in the pathogenesis of inflammatory renal disease or nephritis was first proposed over 80 years ago, and this proposal has subsequently been supported by a wealth of experimental data. Most nephritides are characterized by an inflammatory reaction within the glomerulus accompanied by leucocyte infiltration and cellular proliferation. However, in some forms of nephritis cellular infiltration and proliferation are minimal or even absent. The underlying cause of most nephritides is an antigen–antibody reaction. This reaction may be localized in the glomerulus, antiglomerular antibodies recognizing their target antigen in the tissue, or it may occur remote from the kidney, with subsequent deposition in the glomerulus of immune complexes formed elsewhere in the circulation. In either case, antibody immobilized in the glomerulus will initiate inflammation by activating complement and recruiting inflammatory cells. The different clinical features and pathologies in the various forms of nephritis are dictated by the precise anatomical location and quantity of antigen–antibody complex deposition in the glomerulus, and by the nature of the constituents — in particular, the type of immunoglobulin — in the complex.

Although numerous effector mechanisms, including T cells, cytokines and prostaglandins, have been implicated in the pathogenesis of nephritis it remains clear that complement plays a central role. This chapter concentrates on this role of complement in the various types of nephritis. It should be emphasized at this stage that complement activation is in most cases just one aspect, albeit an important one, of the immune reaction in the glomerulus. For accounts of the involvement of other effector mechanisms the reader is referred to the list at the end of this chapter.

The many elegant animal models of nephritis which have been developed have provided a wealth of experimental data and invaluable insights into the pathogeneses of the human diseases they resemble. These models, and the role of complement in them, are described in the first section of this chapter. Evidence for similar mechanisms in human nephritis is presented in later sections.

## 6.2 ANIMAL MODELS OF HUMAN NEPHRITIS

Experimental models of nephritis were first described over 90 years ago. Immunization of rats with antikidney antibodies caused renal disease, although at that time no human equivalent of this model disease was recognized. Subsequent attempts to induce nephritis in experimental animals have involved immunization with a variety of renal and nonrenal antigens and injection of diverse antibodies against glomerular antigens. From these studies several 'benchmark' models have emerged which have been reproducible in different laboratories and whose pathologies resemble those of specific human diseases. However, as with all animal models, extrapolations to human disease should be made with caution.

Complement involvement in pathogenesis has been investigated by using animals deficient in specific complement components or by artificially depleting complement using cobra venom factor (CVF), a C3b-like protein isolated from cobra venom. After injection into the animal CVF binds Factor B to form a very stable C3 convertase (half-life about 8 hours) which rapidly consumes all the available C3, rendering the animal complement deficient for up to 5 days. The important models and the evidence for an involvement of complement in them are discussed below.

### 6.2.1 Serum sickness glomerulonephritis

Serum sickness glomerulonephritis is induced in rabbits by immunization with bovine serum albumin (BSA). Acute and chronic variants of the disease can be induced by altering the amount of antigen and the frequency of immunization. Immune complexes containing BSA and anti-BSA antibodies are formed in the circulation and become deposited in the glomerulus, predominantly in the glomerular capillary wall. The disease is the classical model of an immune complex disease. In the chronic form, proliferative changes occur in the glomerulus and aggregates of IgG and C3 are present along glomerular capillary walls. Membrane attack complexes (MACs) are also present in the glomerulus, providing evidence that activation of the complement system has continued to completion. MACs are present in subepithelial dense deposits, on the epithelial cell foot processes and on the basement membrane, and it has been suggested that this cytotoxic complex is, at least in part, responsible for the basement membrane damage and epithelial cell injury which result in proteinuria. In its acute form serum sickness glomerulonephritis resembles the human disease acute poststreptococcal nephritis and in its chronic form shares some features with the nephritis of systemic lupus erythematosus (SLE) (see Section 6.3).

### 6.2.2 Anti-GBM nephritis

Anti-GBM nephritis is induced in experimental animals by injection of heterologous antibodies directed against the glomerular basement membrane (GBM). In the early stages, antibody binds in a linear pattern along the endothelial or vascular surface of the basement membrane and induces a proliferative nephritis. The human counterpart of anti-GBM nephritis is *Goodpasture's syndrome*, a rare nephritis which, like the experimental disease, is characterized by linear deposition of immunoglobulin on the basement membrane.

In anti-GBM nephritis, activation of complement releases chemotactic factors which recruit phagocytes into the glomerulus and establish a typical inflammatory reaction. In the later, autologous phase of the disease the animal produces antibody against the heterologous immunoglobulin, which binds to fixed immunoglobulin in the glomerulus, exacerbating the inflammation. Although complement is important in the causation of glomerular infiltration in this model there is evidence that, at least in some species, infiltrating T cells are central to the pathogenesis of glomerular injury. However, induction of anti-GBM nephritis in the rabbit requires an intact complement system, C6-deficient animals being refractory to disease. This observation firmly implicates the MAC in the pathogenesis of this variant of the disease (for details of these studies, see the papers by Salant and coworkers listed at the end of this chapter).

### 6.2.3 Heymann nephritis

Heymann nephritis is induced in rats by immunization with kidney homogenates (active) or by injection of heterologous antibodies against glomerular antigens (passive). On clinical and histological grounds Heymann nephritis resembles human *membranous nephropathy*. The experimental disease is characterized histologically by finely granular subepithelial deposits of IgG and C3, with little glomerular proliferation or cellular infiltration (Fig. 6.1). The lack of infiltration is probably due to the location of the immune deposits on the side of the GBM remote from the vascular space, which prevents neutrophil recruitment by released chemotactic agents. Activation of complement in the subepithelial space has been implicated in the disruption of the glomerular permeability barrier which occurs in this disease and results in severe proteinuria.

Passive Heymann nephritis (PHN), induced in rats by injection of antibodies against the brush border of the proximal tubules, is one of the most studied animal models of nephritis and has provided much information on the likely mechanisms by which deposition of immune complexes causes glomerular injury. It has been known for some years that glomerular injury in this model is dependent on the presence of an intact complement system but independent of neutrophil infiltration. More recently the mechanisms of complement damage have become better defined. In both the experimental disease and human membranous nephritis deposition of MACs in the damaged glomeruli has been demonstrated (Fig. 6.1). Definitive proof of an involvement of the MAC in the pathogenesis of PHN has been provided by studies using an isolated perfused rat kidney variant of the PHN model. Perfusion of the antibody-treated kidney with serum resulted in proteinuria. If C8-deficient serum was used proteinuria was absent, but addition of C8 to the deficient serum restored the effect. As the only known role of C8 is to participate in the formation of the cytopathic MAC, these findings provide strong evidence that the MAC is a major pathogenic factor in this model (see papers by Salant *et al.* and by Couser *et al.* listed at the end of this chapter).

### 6.2.4 Anti-TBM nephritis

Immunization of experimental animals with homologous or heterologous tubular basement membranes (TBM) or injection of anti-TBM antibodies results in a nephritis involving primarily the proximal

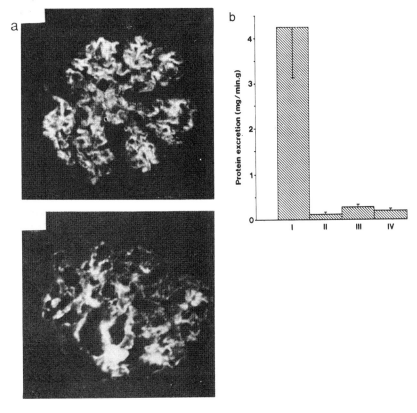

*Figure 6.1* Complement in Heymann nephritis.
(a) Sections from isolated perfused rat kidney treated with antiglomerular antibody and complement to produce nephritis: staining for IgG (*top*) or C3 (*bottom*). Magnification × 360. From Cybulsky et al., *J. Clin. Invest.* **77**, 1096–1107 (1986), with permission. (b) Protein excretion from the isolated perfused kidney: I, kidney perfused with anti-glomerular antibody and fresh plasma; II, kidney perfused with antibody and heat-inactivated plasma; III, kidney perfused with antibody plus C8-depleted plasma; IV, kidney perfused with plasma alone. Modified from Cybulsky et al., *Am. J. Physiol.* **129**, 373 (1987).

tubules and kidney interstitium (tubulointerstitial nephritis). The disease is characterized clinically by glucosuria, haematuria, mild proteinuria and uraemia and histologically by deposition of IgG and C3 along the TBM, cellular infiltration and destruction of the proximal tubules. The model disease closely resembles human tubulointerstitial nephritis, although this latter disease is remarkably heterogeneous. An involvement of complement, and specifically the alternative pathway, in the pathogenesis of anti-TBM nephritis is suggested by the finding of C3 and Factor B, but not C4, along the TBM. Animals depleted of complement using CVF are refractory to disease but TBM nephritis can be induced in animals deficient in C4, again implicating the alternative pathway. The infiltrating phagocytic cells, which are attracted to the area by complement-derived factors, are also required for disease expression, indicating that multiple pathogenic factors are involved.

### 6.2.5 Complement and animal models of nephritis

The important animal models of nephritis, their human disease counterparts and the evidence for complement involvement are summarized in Table 6.1. Complement may be involved directly or indirectly in pathogenesis. Neutrophil accumulation at the inflammatory site is mediated largely by activation of complement which attracts neutrophils from the circulation (C3a, C5a, C5adesArg), traps them in the tissues (immune adherence to fixed C3b) and stimulates them to release toxic mediators (C5a, MAC). Release of these toxic molecules from neutrophils in close proximity to the GBM will cause degradation of the barrier. Complement may also be involved directly in disrupting the permeability barrier. The major pathogenic factor here is likely to be the MAC, which can damage or destroy glomerular epithelial cells and form large pores in the GBM.

*Table 6.1* Animal models of nephritis.

| Type | Complement involvement | Human equivalent |
|---|---|---|
| Serum sickness | C3, MAC in glomerulus | Poststreptococcal nephritis |
| Anti-GBM nephritis | C3 in glomerulus; C6 deficiency protects (rabbit) | Goodpasture's syndrome |
| Heymann nephritis | C3, MAC in glomerulus; C8 depletion protects | Membranous nephropathy |
| Anti-TBM nephritis | C3, FB along TBM; C depletion protects | Tubulointerstitial nephritis |
| IgA nephropathy | C3 in glomerulus | IgA nephropathy |
| Murine SLE | C3 in glomerulus; systemic C activation | SLE nephropathy |

C, complement; MAC, membrane attack complex; FB, Factor B.

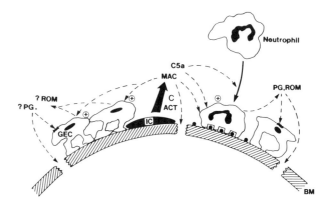

*Figure 6.2* Mechanisms of complement-mediated glomerular injury.
Immune complexes (IC) in the glomerulus activate complement, leading to the production of active molecules, including C5a and the MAC. C5a attracts neutrophils into the glomerulus where they bind via receptors to C3b (●) on the basement membrane (BM). C5a and the MAC have cytopathic and stimulatory effects on infiltrating neutrophils and on glomerular epithelial cells (GECs), causing the release of inflammatory mediators which may in turn damage glomerular cells or the BM. PG, prostaglandins; ROM, reactive oxygen metabolites.

The mechanisms by which complement may contribute to pathogenesis in experimental nephritis are summarized in Fig. 6.2.

### 6.3 COMPLEMENT AND HUMAN NEPHRITIS

Evidence for the participation of complement in human nephritis has been obtained indirectly by the demonstration of decreased serum levels of total complement activity or of individual components, or increased levels of the products of complement activation (see Chapter 12). More direct evidence is provided by the immunohistochemical detection of complement components within the diseased kidney. It is obviously not possible to manipulate the complement system in man in the ways described in the preceding section, making it more difficult to obtain convincing evidence of a pathogenic role of complement. Nevertheless, cautious extrapolation from animal models together with measurements of fluid-phase and tissue complement provide a basis for implicating complement in several human nephritides.

Congenital deficiency of complement, particularly of the early components, is associated with immune complex disease, the commonest manifestation of which is nephritis. This association occurs because of the importance of complement in maintaining immune complexes in a soluble state (see Section 2.4). Thus under different circumstances complement activation can be protective or pathological. Complement protects against immune complex deposition in the kidney by maintaining complexes in solution. If, however, complexes are formed *in situ*, or are deposited despite solubilization, complement activation within the kidney contributes to inflammation and tissue damage.

The following sections describe the contribution of complement to pathogenesis in selected renal diseases. It is not the intention to provide an account of the role of complement in every renal disease but rather to give examples of its pathological importance. Table 6.2 lists the renal diseases in which complement has been implicated and summarizes the evidence for its involvement.

*Table 6.2* Complement in human nephritis.

| Disease | Evidence for complement involvement |
| --- | --- |
| Acute poststreptococcal nephritis | Systemic hypocomplementaemia ( ↓ ↓ C3, ↓ C4, ↓ C2); glomerular deposits of C3, C4, C2, MAC |
| IgA nephropathy | Systemic hypocomplementaemia ( ↓ C3, ↓ FB); glomerular deposits of C3, properdin, MAC |
| Membranous nephropathy | Systemic hypocomplementaemia ( ↓ C3); glomerular deposits of C3, MAC |
| Membranoproliferative GN Type I | Glomerular deposits of C3, C1, C4 |
| Membranoproliferative GN Type II | Systemic hypocomplementaemia ( ↓ C3, ↓ FB); glomerular deposits of C3 |
| Membranoproliferative GN Type III | Systemic hypocomplementaemia ( ↓ C5–C9); glomerular deposits of C3, C5, properdin, MAC |
| Goodpasture's syndrome | Glomerular deposits of C3 (50%) |
| SLE nephritis | Systemic hypocomplementaemia ( ↓ C3, ↓ C4, ↓ C2); glomerular deposits of C3, MAC |
| Tubulointerstitial nephritis | Peritubular deposits of C3 |

MAC, membrane attack complex; FB, Factor B; GN, glomerular nephritis.

## 6.3.1 Complement and IgA nephropathy

IgA nephropathy (Berger's disease) presents in children and young adults with recurrent haematuria, often following a respiratory infection. A proportion of patients develop progressive disease leading to renal failure. IgA nephropathy may also be associated with a number of diseases, including Henoch–Schönlein purpura and hepatic failure. Pathologically the disease is characterized by diffuse deposits of IgA in the mesangium of all glomeruli and by mesangial proliferation. C3 and properdin, but not C4 and C2, are present in close association with the IgA deposits, suggesting predominant alternative pathway activation. Widespread mesangial deposition of the MAC has also recently been demonstrated, and a role for the MAC in glomerular damage proposed (Fig. 6.3). In the serum, IgA levels are raised and in the acute stages, total haemolytic complement activity is reduced, implying activation. Alternative-pathway component depletion predominates, confirming that most complement activation in this disease occurs via the alternative pathway.

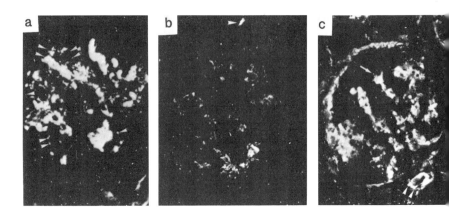

*Figure 6.3* Complement in IgA nephropathy.
Sections of renal tissue from patients with IgA nephropathy. (*a*) Extensive granular deposits of IgA in the glomerulus identified by immunofluorescence. (*b*) Immunofluorescence localization of the membrane attack complex (MAC) predominantly in the mesangium. (*c*) MAC deposition in the mesangium and at the periphery of the glomerulus. Magnification × 125. Reproduced from Rauterberg *et al.*, *Kidney Int.* **31**, 820–829 (1987), with permission.

### 6.3.2 Acute poststreptococcal nephritis

Poststreptococcal nephritis is a rare sequela of streptococcal infections of the throat or skin. About 2–3 weeks after the infective episode patients present with haematuria and proteinuria which in a minority may develop into nephrotic syndrome or acute renal failure. Although most make a full recovery, a few may progress to chronic renal failure. The disease clinically and pathologically resembles experimental serum sickness nephritis induced in animals by immunization with large amounts of foreign protein (Section 6.2.1).

Within the kidney there is a proliferative glomerulonephritis accompanied by granular deposits of immunoglobulin and complement. Measurement of serum complement reveals profound hypocomplementaemia, with low levels of C3 and usually of C4 and C2. The severity of the hypocomplementaemia is out of proportion to the amount of complement fixation occurring in the kidney, implying that activation may also be taking place at other sites. In some individuals an autoantibody is present in the serum, the C4 nephritic factor, which stabilizes the C4b2a complex, enhancing complement activation.

### 6.3.3 Membranoproliferative glomerulonephritis (MPGN) Type II

MPGN Type II predominantly affects young adults who present with severe proteinuria, often accompanied by haematuria and progressive renal failure. Dense deposits of immunoglobulin and C3 are present in the glomeruli and tubules, mainly on the basement membranes. Patients usually have hypocomplementaemia with low levels of C3 but normal levels of C2 and C4, suggesting alternative pathway activation. The disease is commonly associated with an autoantibody, the C3 nephritic factor (C3NeF), in the serum which binds to and stabilizes the fluid-phase C3b,Bb complex, resulting in overactivation of the alternative-pathway feedback loop and consumption of C3 (see Section 4.2). Whether the nephritis occurs as a result of abnormal immune complex handling, itself a consequence of secondary complement deficiency, or is due to C3NeF localization and complement activation within the kidney is still not clear, although current evidence favours the latter possibility.

MPGN Type II is occasionally associated with a bizarre disorder of subcutaneous fat called partial lipodystrophy. This condition is characterized by the sudden, spontaneous loss of subcutaneous fat from localized areas of the face, arms or trunk. The disease usually presents in childhood following a trivial infection, often measles. In the majority of patients C3NeF is present in the circulation and complement levels are reduced. Months or years later many of these individuals develop MPGN Type II.

### 6.3.4 Membranoproliferative glomerulonephritis (MPGN) Type III

MPGN Type III, though clinically similar to MPGN Type II, is pathologically distinct. Glomerular deposits are more widespread, being present in the mesangium as well as in subendothelial and subepithelial locations, and there is marked disruption of the GBM. The deposits contain C3, C5 and properdin. Systemic hypocomplementaemia is common but the profile reveals decreased levels only of terminal components (C5–C9). Terminal complement activation in MPGN Type III appears to be mediated by an immunoglobulin nephritic factor distinct from that involved in MPGN Type II, which stabilizes the C3 and C5 convertases of the alternative pathway (Section 4.3.5).

### 6.3.5 Membranous nephropathy

Membranous nephropathy presents in adults with proteinuria which may be sufficiently severe to cause the nephrotic syndrome. In the majority the disease is slowly progressive, occasionally leading to renal failure. Circulating immune complexes are absent or present at low levels and serum complement levels are normal. In the kidney immune complexes are detected in the glomeruli in a characteristic subepithelial position. Glomerular infiltration and proliferation are absent. C3 and the MAC can be found by immunohistochemical staining in the glomerular deposits. The possibility of an involvement of complement in pathogenesis is strengthened by the similarities between this condition and the experimental disease Heymann nephritis, in which damage appears to be mediated by the MAC (Section 6.2.3).

## 6.4 COMPLEMENT AND SYSTEMIC LUPUS ERYTHEMATOSUS (SLE)

Systemic lupus erythematosus (SLE) is a chronic, non-organ-specific autoimmune disease affecting primarily the kidneys, joints and skin, although other organs are often involved. More has been written concerning the association between the complement system and SLE than for any other disease, and complement has been implicated in the pathogenesis of tissue damage in many diverse organs in this disease. To provide a concise account of complement in SLE and to prevent repetition, this section describes all aspects of SLE and is not restricted to renal disease.

SLE usually presents in young adults. It is 5–10 times more common in women than in men. The typical clinical presentation includes fever, weight loss, arthralgia, a characteristic butterfly rash and nephritis, although many individuals present with very atypical symptoms. Serologically the disease is associated with the presence of circulating autoantibodies and immune complexes. In most instances the initiation of organ damage can be attributed to the deposition of immune complexes in the tissues. Complement activation in SLE was first documented almost 40 years ago. Serum whole complement activity ($CH_{50}$) and the levels of classical-pathway components are reduced secondary to chronic activation by immune complexes, the extent of this reduction mirroring disease activity, and terminal complement complexes are present in the serum. Measurement of complement activation therefore provides important clinical information on the course of disease and its response to therapy (Table 6.3; for methods of assessing activation, see Section 12.2).

*Table 6.3* Complement profile in SLE.

---

*Idiopathic SLE*
  Systemic hypocomplementaemia (classical and alternative);
  ↓ C4, C1, C2, C3, C5–C9; ↑ TCC; ↓ FB

*Complement-deficiency SLE*
  Systemic hypocomplementaemia (classical only);
  ↓↓ C2, C4 *or* C1; other components normal; no ↑ TCC

---

TCC, terminal complement complex; FB, Factor B.

### 6.4.1 Renal disease and SLE

Renal involvement is found in over one-half of SLE patients, although in most the disease is mild. Some individuals develop an acute nephritis which can rapidly progress to renal failure, while others present with severe proteinuria and the nephrotic syndrome. Even those with mild renal disease may eventually develop chronic nephritis and renal failure. Immunohistological investigations have provided abundant evidence of an involvement of complement in SLE. Immune complexes and C3 are present in association with the glomerular basement membrane (GBM) and in glomerular capillaries, and the MAC is found in glomeruli and proximal and distal tubules in close proximity to areas of disrupted basement membrane, implicating this complex in renal damage (Fig. 6.4). The extent of immunoglobulin and complement (particularly MAC) deposition is related to the severity of renal impairment.

### 6.4.2 Joint disease and SLE

More than 90% of patients with SLE complain of pains in their joints during the course of their disease. Less commonly, individuals have a true arthritis with inflammation and redness. Joint destruction of the type seen in rheumatoid arthritis is rare in SLE. Immune complexes and complement are present in the synovial membrane of

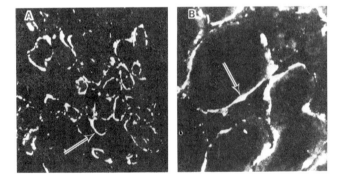

*Figure 6.4* MAC deposition in SLE nephritis.
The MAC is localized by immunofluorescence in renal tissue in SLE. The figure shows prominent peritubular staining in the region of the tubular basement membrane (arrowed). Magnification: (A) × 150; (B) × 400. Reproduced from Biesecker, *Lab. Invest.* **49**, 237–249 (1983), with permission.

the inflamed joint, the synovial fluid contains immune complexes and synovial fluid complement levels are usually markedly diminished, providing evidence of complement activation in the joint. Activation complexes and individual components have not been measured in the joints in SLE.

### 6.4.3 Skin disease and SLE

The classical skin lesion of SLE, the 'butterfly rash' on the cheeks and bridge of the nose, is only one of the diverse dermatological symptoms associated with SLE. Erythematous rashes may occur elsewhere on the body, and healing with scaling produces so-called *discoid* lesions. Biopsies of lesional skin show deposits of immunoglobulin, C3 and the MAC at the dermal–epidermal junction. Immunoglobulin and C3, but not the MAC, are also often found in apparently normal skin in SLE. In lesions the MAC is located on basement membranes and cell membranes, and may directly damage these structures directly or indirectly.

### 6.4.4 Neurological disease and SLE

About one-third of individuals with SLE have evidence of neurological involvement which may manifest itself as behavioural disturbances or frank psychosis, or as organic brain disease with convulsions or, rarely, paralysis. Central nervous system (CNS) involvement has been reported to be second only to renal failure as a cause of death in SLE. Measurement of C4 levels in the cerebrospinal fluid (CSF) of patients with SLE with or without CNS involvement has revealed a strong association between the presence and severity of CNS involvement and decreased levels of C4, suggesting that complement is activated in the CNS. More recently this suggestion has been supported by the demonstration that levels of the terminal complement complex are increased in the CSF of SLE patients with CNS involvement, and a pathogenic role for complement has been proposed.

### 6.4.5 Complement deficiency and SLE

As described in Chapter 4, a majority of individuals with deficiencies of components of the classical pathway, specifically C1, C4 and

C2, present with SLE or an SLE-like illness, although it should be emphasized that the great majority of patients with SLE do not have an inherited complement deficiency. Well over 100 individuals have been described who have SLE and a deficiency of one of these components (Table 4.2), most being deficient in C2. Deficiency of C3 may also give rise to SLE but more commonly presents with severe, recurrent infections. The clinical picture in deficient individuals is similar to that in nondeficient SLE patients, although skin manifestations are more common in the deficient group.

It has been suggested that the association of SLE with deficiencies of C4 and C2 is an epiphenomenon, arising because the genes for these proteins are located in the major histocompatibility complex (MHC). Linkage with an immune response gene within the MHC, the true disease susceptibility gene, would then give rise to the apparent association. This hypothesis accounts for neither the association of C1 and C3 deficiencies with SLE, nor the occurrence of SLE in individuals with acquired deficiencies of C4 or C2, for example in hereditary angioedema (Section 4.2.5). Final proof that it is the complement deficiency itself which is responsible for disease is provided by the successful treatment of SLE in deficient individuals by restoring the missing component. It is probable that SLE occurs in complement-deficient individuals because of defective immune complex handling. In the absence of a normal classical pathway the capacity to fix C1 and C3 on immune complexes is diminished or lost. Immune complex solubilization and erythrocyte transport are thus impaired, resulting in the formation of insoluble complexes which precipitate in the tissues (Section 2.4). Thus, in both the complement-deficient and complement-sufficient individual with SLE, disease occurs because of deposition of immune complexes in the tissues. In the former case deposition occurs because of an inability to handle the normal immune complex load, whereas in the latter it is the result of a greatly increased immune complex load which overwhelms normal handling mechanisms (Fig. 6.5).

Partial deficiency of C4, specifically of the isotype C4A, may also be associated with SLE. Following activation C4A binds to amino groups on surfaces whereas C4B binds to hydroxyl groups. Defective handling of immune complexes bearing predominantly amino groups therefore occurs in C4A deficient individuals and is likely to be responsible for disease. Both homozygous and heterozygous C4A deficiencies are common amongst patients with SLE but the association will be missed without specialist investigation as

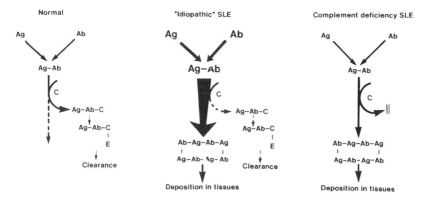

*Figure 6.5* Immune complex handling in SLE.
In the normal situation, immune complexes (Ag–Ab) activate complement (C), become coated with C3b, and are thus kept small and soluble. Complement-containing immune complexes bind to erythrocytes (E) and are thereby removed from the circulation. In idiopathic SLE, increased immune complex formation saturates the solubilizing capacity of a normal complement system, resulting in deposition of complexes in the tissues. In complement-deficiency SLE, absence of a classical pathway component prevents activation, allowing large, insoluble complexes to form.

immunochemical measurements of C4 reveal low normal levels, a common finding in idiopathic SLE (Table 6.3).

### 6.4.6 Complement receptors and SLE

The association between complement receptors and SLE has attracted much attention in recent years. The C3b/C4b receptor $CR_1$ plays an important role in immune complex clearance and it is clear that erythrocytes from patients with SLE have decreased numbers of $CR_1$ on their surfaces and that receptor number is related to disease activity. Two allelles for $CR_1$ exist, coding for high or low receptor number, and it has been suggested that inheritance of low $CR_1$ number predisposes to SLE. However, careful examination of inheritance patterns provides strong evidence that low numbers of $CR_1$ on SLE erythrocytes are an acquired characteristic. Erythrocytes with high $CR_1$ number rapidly lose receptors when transfused into an individual with SLE, confirming that the deficiency is acquired. The mechanism of $CR_1$ loss is not known but is likely to be related to erythrocyte immune complex processing.

### 6.4.7 Drug-induced SLE

It has been known for many years that some commonly used drugs can rarely, after long-term use, induce a disease condition which closely resembles SLE. The drugs include the antihypertensive hydralazine, the antitubercle agent isoniazid, and penicillamine, which is used in the treatment of severe rheumatoid arthritis. The mechanism by which these drugs induce SLE has recently been established. All three drugs inhibit binding of activated C4b to surfaces by interacting with the nascent thiolester site exposed upon cleavage of C4 (see Fig. 1.4). Failure of C4b to bind to forming immune complexes results in defective handling of complexes and deposition in the tissues. The drugs interact much more avidly with the C4A isotype than with C4B. As discussed above (Section 6.4.5), individuals who have a homozygous or even heterozygous deficiency of C4A are at increased risk of developing idiopathic SLE. Because of the differential effects of these C4-inhibiting drugs, individuals with heterozygous deficiency of C4A are also much more vulnerable to drug-induced SLE.

### 6.5. COMPLEMENT AND RENAL DISEASE

From the above account it is clear that complement is implicated in many renal diseases. Its relative contribution to the overall pathology is difficult to assess and it is clear that in most of these diseases complement is just one of several interacting pathogenic forces. Without doubt, the major role of complement with respect to renal (and other immune-complex-mediated) disease is a protective one, maintaining immune complexes in solution and solubilizing precipitated complexes. The importance of this is illustrated graphically in individuals with congenital or acquired deficiencies of complement. Activation of complement in the tissues will, however, produce toxic mediators which can cause tissue damage indirectly or directly. The demonstration that formation of the MAC is necessary for disease expression in some animal models of nephritis raises the intriguing possibility that specific inhibition of the MAC — without interfering with the activation pathways responsible for immune complex solubilization — might be of therapeutic value in human nephritis.

## 6.6 FURTHER READING

*Animal models*

Brentjens, J. R., Noble, B. and Andres, G. A. (1982). Immunologically mediated lesions of kidney tubules and interstitium in laboratory animals and man. *Springer Semin. Immunopathol.* **5**, 357–378.

Cochrane, C. G. (1984). The role of complement in experimental disease models. *Springer Semin. Immunopathol.* **7**, 263–270.

Salant, D. J., Quigg, R. J. and Cybulsky, A. V. (1989). Heymann nephritis: mechanisms of renal injury. *Kidney Int.* **35**, 976–984.

Hoedemaeker, P. J. and Weening, J. J. (1989). Relevance of experimental models for human nephropathology. *Kidney Int.* **35**, 1015–1025.

*Human disease*

Schreiber, R. D. and Müller-Eberhard, H. J. (1979). Complement and renal disease. In: Wilson, C. B., Brewer, B. M. and Stein, J. M. (eds), *Contemporary Issues in Nephrology*, Vol. 3. Churchill Livingstone, Edinburgh, pp. 67–105.

Williams, D. G. and Peters, D. K. (1982). The immunology of nephritis. In: Lachmann, P. J. and Peters, D. K. (eds), *Clinical Aspects of Immunology*, Vol. 2. Blackwell, Oxford, pp. 853–877.

Couser, W. G., Baker, P. J. and Adler, S. (1985). Complement and the direct mediation of immune glomerular injury: a new perspective. *Kidney Int.* **28**, 879–890.

Couser, W. G. (1985). Mechanisms of glomerular injury in immune complex disease. *Kidney Int.* **28**, 569–583.

Rauterberg, E. W., Lieberknecht, H. M., Wingen, A. M. and Ritz, E. (1987). Complement membrane attack (MAC) in idiopathic IgA-glomerulonephritis. *Kidney Int.* **31**, 820–829.

*SLE*

Schur, P. H. (1982). Complement and lupus erythematosus. *Arthritis Rheum.* **25**, 793–798.

Atkinson, J. P. (1986). Complement activation and complement receptors in systemic lupus erythematosus. *Springer Semin. Immunopathol.* **9**, 179–194.

Sim, E. (1989). Drug-induced immune complex disease. *Complement Inflamm.* **6**, 119–128.

Lachmann, P. J. (1990) Complement deficiency and the pathogenesis of autoimmune immune complex. In: Waksman, B. H. (ed.) *1939–1989: Fifty Years Progress in Allergy. Chem. Immunol.* Vol. 49. Karger, Basel, pp. 245–263.

CHAPTER SEVEN
# Complement and Rheumatic Disease

## 7.1 INTRODUCTION

Inflammatory rheumatic diseases, like the renal diseases described in the preceding chapter, are mediated predominantly by immune complexes which deposit in the tissues. Complement activation on immune complexes, by maintaining them in solution and by solubilizing complexes which have deposited in the tissues, protects against tissue damage. However, complement activation on precipitated complexes in the tissues releases toxic products which contribute to damage at the site. The protective role of complement is illustrated by the high incidence of rheumatological diseases in individuals deficient in the early components of the classical pathway, C1, C4 or C2. Evidence of a pathogenic role for complement may be obtained by demonstrating disease-related complement consumption and deposition of components in the damaged tissue. The data implicating complement in the arthritis of systemic lupus erythematosus (SLE) were discussed in the previous chapter. Several animal models of inflammatory arthritis have been developed and have provided a means of testing the importance of a variety of potentially pathogenic factors. The first section of this chapter describes these experimental diseases and the role of complement in them. Later sections discuss the contribution of complement activation to tissue damage in human rheumatoid disease.

Most of the experimental and human arthritides are multifactorial, humoral and cellular immune mechanisms and other factors all contributing to damage. This chapter concentrates on the role of complement. For more general accounts of pathogenesis, the reader is referred to the list at the end of this chapter.

## 7.2 COMPLEMENT IN ANIMAL MODELS OF ARTHRITIS

Several animal models of inflammatory arthritis have been developed and have provided valuable insights into disease pathogenesis. The role of complement has been well studied in two of these model diseases, detailed below. Both of these models provide evidence that complement can be involved in the production of joint damage which closely resembles that seen in human inflammatory arthritis. Extrapolation from experimental disease to the human disease must be undertaken only with great caution. Neither of the model systems exactly mimics arthritis in man, and the mechanisms of pathology in human arthritis are complex and multiple. However, taken together with direct evidence from the human diseases, the data obtained in model systems help to establish which of the possible pathogenic factors are important in rheumatoid arthritis (RA) and in other arthritides.

### 7.2.1 Type II collagen-induced arthritis

Type II collagen-induced arthritis is the experimental disease which most closely resembles human RA. It is induced in susceptible strains of rats or mice by intradermal injection of heterologous Type II collagen emulsified in mineral oil. An inflammatory arthritis ensues about 10 days after the injection and causes joint damage which closely resembles that of RA, with cellular infiltration and synovial proliferation which progresses to pannus formation and erosion of joint surfaces. There is abundant evidence that the production of antibodies against the injected protein which cross-react with autologous Type II collagen is responsible for the initiation of disease. The disease can be transferred passively from an actively immunized animal to an unimmunized recipient by transfusion of serum — or purified immunoglobulin — alone. Collagen immunity has also been described in association with RA and other human rheumatic diseases, including polychondritis and systemic sclerosis, making this experimental disease a particularly good model for these conditions.

Evidence for an involvement of complement in the pathogenesis of Type II collagen-induced arthritis was provided initially by examining the effects of decomplementation using cobra venom factor (CVF) (Section 6.2). Whether the disease was induced actively (immunizing with collagen) or passively (serum transfer), animals treated with CVF were refractory to disease until their complement levels recovered. It was shown subsequently that C5-deficient mice are also resistant to the induction of active or passive disease, implicating C5 activation, and thus C5a or MAC production, in disease pathogenesis.

### 7.2.2 Acute allergic arthritis

Acute allergic arthritis is induced in rabbits by first immunizing with an antigen (commonly bovine serum albumin) in Freund's complete adjuvant (mineral oil containing killed mycobacteria), followed 2–3 weeks later by an intra-articular injection of the same antigen. An inflammatory synovitis develops in the injected joint, with pronounced cellular infiltration and synovial proliferation. Pannus formation and erosions occur in the joint, the overall pathology closely resembling that of RA. The arthritis is usually chronic, persisting for years following a single intra-articular injection. The inflamed synovium contains many plasma cells which produce antibodies, about one-third of which are directed against the original antigen. Interaction of these antibodies with antigen produces immune complexes which deposit in the synovium and activate complement.

Evidence of an involvement of complement in the pathogenesis of this disease has again been provided by utilizing complement-depleted or complement-deficient animals. Decomplementation with CVF prior to intra-articular injection of antigen inhibits cellular infiltration and disease expression. Rabbits deficient in C6 are refractory to disease, implicating the MAC in the development of clinical symptoms.

### 7.3 COMPLEMENT IN HUMAN ARTHRITIS

It is obviously not possible to decomplement humans acutely in order to obtain evidence of a role of complement in disease pathogenesis. Evidence implicating complement may, however, be provided by demonstrating systemic or localized complement activation and deposition of complement fragments in diseased tissues, particularly when these parameters closely mirror disease activity.

### 7.3.1 Complement and rheumatoid arthritis

Rheumatoid arthritis is a common chronic inflammatory disease of unknown aetiology which affects principally the joints. It is two to three times more frequent in females and usually involves the small joints of the hands and wrists. Involved joints become swollen, hot and painful, and joint destruction often ensues. Up to 90% of patients with RA have an IgM autoantibody reactive with the Fc portion of IgG in their serum: this is termed rheumatoid factor.

Within the inflamed joint the synovial membrane is thickened, a consequence both of synovial cell proliferation and infiltration with inflammatory cells, including T and B lymphocytes and macrophages. Fluid containing large numbers of inflammatory cells accumulates in the joint space, and immune complexes, a proportion of which incorporate rheumatoid factor, are present in the fluid and within the synovial membrane. These complexes can activate complement and stimulate phagocytic cells directly, thus amplifying the inflammatory response in the joint (Fig. 7.1). The nature of the antigen responsible for initiating the process remains uncertain, although a variety of microorganisms, including mycobacteria, have been implicated.

Although there is abundant evidence implicating complement activation in RA, systemic hypocomplementaemia is not a common feature, most patients having normal or even elevated serum complement levels. This finding is a consequence of the localized nature of inflammation in RA, increased consumption in the joint being compensated — or overcompensated — for by increased synthesis. Diminished serum complement levels are occasionally found during acute exacerbations of the disease when demand temporarily outstrips supply. Systemic evidence of complement utilization is provided by measurement of the products of activation. The fragments C3d and C3dg, the terminal complement complex (TCC) and the C1/C1inh complex are present in serum at levels which correlate well with each other and with disease activity (Fig. 7.2, Table 7.1).

In the synovial fluid, complement activity is usually reduced, reflecting the intense local activation. Levels of C3 and C4 are often

## 134  Complement and Rheumatic Disease

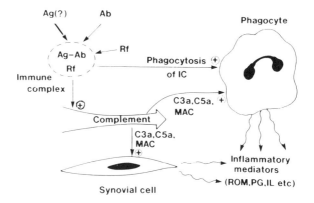

*Figure 7.1* Complement and inflammation in the rheumatoid joint.
Immune complexes (Ag–Ab), often including rheumatoid factor (Rf), are formed in the joint and activate complement via the classical and perhaps also the alternative pathways. Complement chemotactic factors (C3a, C5a) attract phagocytic cells into the joint. Phagocytes are activated by complement products (C3a, C5a and the MAC) and also by phagocytosis of immune complexes to release a variety of pro-inflammatory molecules, including reactive oxygen metabolites (ROM), prostaglandins (PG) and interleukins (IL). Complement products may also stimulate synovial cells to release inflammatory mediators.

low but measurement of breakdown products again provides a much better assessment of complement turnover. Fragments of C3, C4 and Factor B, and the C1/C1inh and TCC activation complexes, are present in the synovial fluid at levels which reflect disease activity (Table 7.1). The presence of both the C1/C1inh complex and split products of Factor B indicates that complement activation occurs via both the classical and alternative activation pathways, and the presence of TCCs implies that the terminal pathway is also activated to completion in the joint.

Further evidence of complement involvement has been provided by the demonstration of complement components and activation products in the synovial membrane. C3 and C4 are deposited diffusely in the membrane and the MAC is present particularly at the borders of the membrane and in the walls of small blood vessels. The MAC has also been demonstrated in the synovial fluid on small membrane fragments or vesicles which are presumably derived from synovial cells or inflammatory cells in the joint (Fig. 7.3). This finding has stimulated the proposal that the cells in the inflamed synovium are subjected to chronic, low-level complement membrane attack, but resist lysis and recover by shedding MACs from their

Table 7.1 Complement profile in active rheumatoid arthritis.

|  | Serum | Synovial fluid |
|---|---|---|
| $CH_{50}$ | N or ↑ | ↓ ↓ |
| C3 | N or ↑ | ↓ |
| C4 | N or ↑ | ↓ |
| C3d(dg) | ++ | +++ |
| C9 | ↑ | ↑ |
| C1/C1inh | ++ | +++ |
| TCC | ++ | +++ |

N, normal (all levels relative to control fluids from individuals without inflammatory disease).

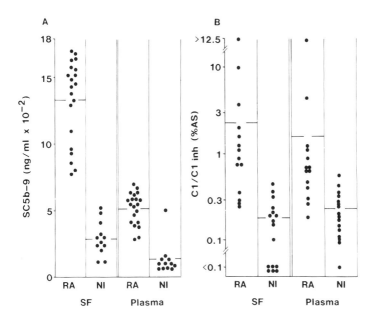

Figure 7.2 Terminal complement complex and C1/C1inh complex levels in rheumatoid arthritis.

The fluid-phase terminal complement complex (SC5b–9) (A) and the C1/C1 inhibitor complex (B) measured in paired samples of plasma and synovial fluid (SF) from patients with rheumatoid arthritis (RA) or with noninflammatory joint disease (NI) by ELISA assay. Horizontal bars in each column represent means. (A) Modified from Morgan et al., Clin. Exp. Immunol. **73**, 473–478 (1988), with permission. (B) Data by courtesy of Dr D. A. Oleesky, Cardiff.

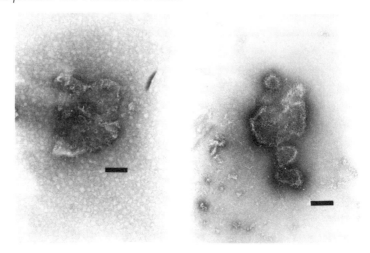

*Figure 7.3* MAC-bearing membrane fragments in rheumatoid synovial fluid. Transmission electron micrographs of membrane fragments (vesicles?) isolated from rheumatoid synovial fluid. The fragments are covered with ring-like lesions having the typical appearance of the MAC. Scale bar in each micrograph represents 100 nm. From Morgan *et al.*, *Clin. Exp. Immunol.* **73**, 467–472 (1988), with permission.

surfaces, as described in other cell types (Section 1.3.3.4). *In vitro*, complement activation — and specifically nonlethal membrane attack — has been shown to stimulate rheumatoid synovial cells to release toxic mediators including reactive oxygen metabolites and prostaglandins. These substances may play an important role in propagating inflammation in the joint.

### 7.3.2 Complement and other inflammatory joint diseases

The role of complement in other arthritides has been much less well studied. Many of these diseases are variants of RA, displaying similar joint pathology but having extra-articular manifestations which do not occur in RA. The evidence implicating complement in their pathogenesis is summarized in Table 7.2.

*Juvenile rheumatoid arthritis*, which by definition presents in children under the age of 16 years, differs from the adult disease in that systemic symptoms, including fever and rashes, are common and the joint disease is frequently monoarticular. Measurement of complement activation products in the synovial fluid indicates intra-articular activation but the relevance of this to disease activity is uncertain.

*Sjogren's syndrome* is a variant of RA characterized by decreased

Table 7.2 Complement profile in other inflammatory arthritides.

| | $CH_{50}$ | | Activation products | |
|---|---|---|---|---|
| | Serum | Synovial fluid | Serum | Synovial fluid |
| Juvenile rheumatoid arthritis | N or ↑ | ↓ | +/− | ++ |
| Sjogren's syndrome | ↓ | ↓↓ | +++ | +++ |
| Psoriatic arthropathy | N or ↓ | ↓ | + | +++ |
| Behcet's disease | N | ↓ | + | ++ |
| Reiter's syndrome | N or ↑ | ↑ | ? | ? |
| Gout | N or ↓ | ↓ | ? | ? |

Activation products include some or all of C3d, C3dg, C1/C1inh, TCC (all levels relative to control fluids from individuals without inflammatory disease).

secretion from lacrimal and salivary glands. Systemic hypocomplementaemia is much more common in this syndrome than it is in RA, suggesting enhanced complement activation. Individuals with low complement levels frequently have cryoglobulinaemia and vasculitis (see below), but local complement activation has not been investigated in this syndrome and the role of complement in the causation of extra-articular pathology has not been examined.

About 5% of patients with psoriasis develop a chronic arthritis. This *psoriatic arthritis* is distinct from RA in that it commonly affects the small joints of the fingers and toes. Complement activation products are present systemically and in the synovial fluid, and the MAC has been localized in the synovial membrane in psoriatic arthritis. The level of activation appears to exceed that found in RA, suggesting that complement may be particularly relevant to pathogenesis in this disease.

*Behcet's disease* is a multisystem disorder characterized by oral and genital ulceration and ocular inflammation. Most patients have arthralgia and many develop a nonerosive polyarthritis. Systemic hypocomplementaemia is not a feature of Behcet's disease but the serum level of complement component C9 is markedly elevated and has been shown to be a sensitive index of disease activity (Fig. 7.4). Increased C9 concentration occurs as part of the acute phase response and does not directly implicate complement in pathogenesis. However, TCCs and membrane fragments or vesicles containing MACs have been identified in serum and synovial fluid from patients with this disease, suggesting a role of complement in tissue damage.

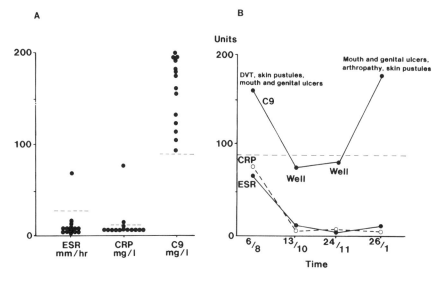

*Figure 7.4* C9 in Behcet's disease.
(*A*) C9, erythrocyte sedimentation rate (ESR), and C-reactive protein (CRP) measured in plasma from patients with Behcet's disease. Dotted line represents upper limit of normal for each measurement. (*B*) C9, CRP and ESR measured at intervals in patients with Behcet's disease and their relationship to clinically assessed disease activity: data for one representative patient. Horizontal, dotted line represents upper limit of normal for C9. Modified from Rumfeld *et al., Brit. J. Rheumatol.* **25**, 266–270 (1986), with permission.

## 7.4 COMPLEMENT AND VASCULITIC SYNDROMES

Inflammation and tissue destruction affecting predominantly the blood vessels are a feature of many diseases, including *polyarteritis nodosa, polymyositis* and *systemic sclerosis*. These diseases are mediated primarily by immune complex deposition in the vessel wall. The initiating antigen in most forms of vasculitis is unknown but viral infections have been implicated in a few instances. Classical-pathway activation on the immune complexes initiates inflammation which may damage or destroy the vessel. Because of the localized nature of the complement activation, systemic hypocomplement-aemia is not a common feature in vasculitis, although up to 50% of patients with polyarteritis have decreased serum complement levels. Despite the normal or near-normal total complement activity, serum levels of C4 are frequently low, reflecting activation predominantly of the classical pathway. In most vasculitic syndromes no comprehensive assessment of the complement profile has been made. Deficiency of C2 is frequently associated with vasculitis, often in the absence of evidence of other immune complex disease.

*Table 7.3* Classification of cryoglobulins.

| Type | Component(s) | Disease association | Symptoms |
| --- | --- | --- | --- |
| I (pure monoclonal) | Monoclonal Ig, usually IgM, occasionally IgG; precipitate at high concentration | Malignant disease: myeloma, Waldenstrom's macroglobulin-aemia | Hyperviscosity, vascular purpura, Raynaud's syndrome |
| II (mixed monoclonal) | Monoclonal Ig, usually IgM, anti-IgG antibody, Ig–anti-Ig complexes | Malignant disease: lymphoma, leukaemia, myeloma, etc. | Renal disease, arthritis, vasculitis |
| III (mixed polyclonal) | Polyclonal IgM (RF-like) anti-IgG, Ig–anti-Ig complexes | Idiopathic SLE, RA, chronic infections | Vasculitis, Raynaud's syndrome |

In *cryoglobulinaemia* abnormal immunoglobulin molecules are present in the circulation which, either alone or when incorporated into immune complexes, precipitate from plasma at low temperature. Cryoglobulinaemia is classified into three types, based on the structure of the cryoglobulins involved (Table 7.3). If cryoglobulinaemia is suspected in an individual special precautions must be observed in sample handling in order to prevent complex precipitation and activation of complement *in vitro*. The disease may occur in isolation or may be associated with other immune complex diseases, notably SLE, or with neoplastic disorders. Precipitation of cryoglobulin complexes in the small blood vessels of the skin where the plasma is cooler obstructs the vessels and thus initiates vasculitis. The specific symptoms of cryoglobulinaemia are therefore induced upon exposure to cold and include Raynaud's phenomenon, vascular purpura and even occasionally peripheral artery occlusion and gangrene. Lesions are most commonly observed on the extensor surfaces of the lower leg and forearm.

Renal disease is a frequent accompaniment of cryoglobulinaemia due to precipitation of cryoglobulins, almost always of the Type II mixed variety (Table 7.3), in the glomerulus. As with other forms of vasculitis, classical pathway activation occurs on precipitated complexes. Consequently, C4 levels are low and systemic hypocomplementaemia is usual when the disease is active. In the presence of cryoglobulinaemic nephritis the complement profile typically shows marked hypocomplementaemia, with very low levels of C1, C4 and C2, and slightly lowered C3.

## 7.5 COMPLEMENT AND RHEUMATIC DISEASES

The demonstration of complement consumption in biological fluids and of complement deposition in the affected tissues in human disease and in animal models, together with the ameliorating effect of decomplementation on the model diseases, strongly implicates complement in the pathogenesis of a variety of rheumatic disorders. The initiating factors and copathogens will differ among these diverse diseases but the possibility remains that measures aimed at specifically inhibiting complement activation might be of therapeutic value in many of these conditions.

## 7.6 FURTHER READING

*Animal models*

Cochrane, C. G. (1984). The role of complement in experimental disease models. *Springer Semin. Immunopathol.* **7**, 263–270.

Stuart, J. M., Cremer, M. A., Townes, A. S. and Kang, A. H. (1982). Type II collagen-induced arthritis in rats. *J. Exp. Med.* **155**, 1–16.

*Human disease*

Adinolfi, M., Beck, S. E. and Lehner, T. (1979). Serum levels of acute phase proteins, C9, factor B and lysozyme in Behcet's syndrome and recurrent oral ulceration. In: Lehner, T. and Barnes, C. G. (eds), *Behcet's Syndrome — Clinical and Immunological Features*. Academic Press, London, pp. 107–125.

Atkinson, J. P., Kane, J. L., Holers, V. M. and Chan, A. C. (1986). Complement and the rheumatic diseases. In: Ross, G. D. (ed.), *Immunobiology of the Complement System*. Academic Press, Orlando, pp. 197–211.

George, D. and Glass, D. (1983). Quantitation of the complement proteins in rheumatic disease. *Clin. Rheum. Dis.* **9**, 177–198.

Morgan, B. P., Daniels, R. H. and Williams, B. D. (1988). Measurement of terminal complement complexes in rheumatoid arthritis. *Clin. Exp. Immunol.* **73**, 473–478.

Sanders, M. E., Kopicky, J. A., Wigley, F. M., Shin, M. L., Frank, M. M. and Joiner, K. A. (1986). *J. Rheumatol.* **13**, 1028–1034.

CHAPTER EIGHT
# Complement in Neurological and Muscular Diseases

## 8.1 INTRODUCTION

Tissue damage in many neurological and muscular diseases is mediated, at least in part, by components of the immune system. Both cellular and humoral elements have been implicated and immune complex deposition demonstrated in these diseases. Evidence for a role of complement has thus far been obtained only in a relatively small number of diseases. As with the rheumatoid and renal diseases discussed in the preceding chapters, complement has been implicated by evidence obtained from animal models and by demonstration of complement activation in fluids and diseased tissue. In all these conditions complement is likely to be only one of several immune and nonimmune factors involved in disease pathogenesis. These other factors are not discussed here but are detailed in several reviews listed at the end of this chapter. Because of the diversity of the diseases described, each is accorded a separate section.

## 8.2 COMPLEMENT IN MYASTHENIA GRAVIS

Myasthenia gravis (MG) is a chronic disease characterized by abnormal muscle fatiguability which may be localized or generalized. Eye and facial muscles are most commonly affected, diplopia being a frequent presenting complaint. The disease may occur at any age and is slightly more common in females — particularly among younger individuals. MG is occasionally associated with a tumour of the thymus and in these cases thymectomy may be curative.

It was suggested over 90 years ago that MG was caused by a toxin acting at the motor nerve endplate. Then, in the early 1970s, evidence of a decrease in the number of acetylcholine receptors at the endplate in MG was reported. Much information on the pathogenesis of MG and the mechanisms of receptor loss has been obtained from animal models, and these studies are described first.

### 8.2.1 Animal models for myasthenia gravis

Immunization of experimental animals with acetylcholine receptor (AChR) purified from the electric organ of the electric eel induces an illness which resembles human MG. Anti-AChR antibodies are present in the serum, and the experimental disease (experimental autoimmune myasthenia gravis, EAMG) can be transferred to an unimmunized animal by injection of serum or antibody from a diseased donor. Evidence of the involvement of anti-AChR antibodies in human MG is provided by the demonstration that immunoglobulin from MG patients contains anti-AChR activity and can induce disease when transfused into animals.

Whether actively (immunization with AChR) or passively (transfusion of anti-AChR antibody) induced, EAMG in rats is characterized clinically by muscle weakness and paralysis. At the endplate there are reduced numbers of AChRs, an inflammatory infiltrate and deposition of IgG and C3. The first indication that complement was involved in pathogenesis was provided by examining the effects of decomplementation with cobra venom factor (CVF, Section 6.2). Following treatment with CVF animals are refractory to disease induced actively or passively. In these animals no inflammatory reaction occurs at the endplate and there is no decrease in AChR number. Thus, complement is required for induction of inflammation and receptor loss. Whether this latter change is mediated directly by complement or caused by infiltrating inflammatory cells recruited by complement, was initially uncertain. Definitive evidence of a direct role of complement in receptor loss in EAMG was provided recently by studies which attempted to induce passive EAMG in rats specifically depleted of individual complement components. Rats depleted of C6 by injection of the Fab' fragment of an anti-C6 antibody prior to treatment with anti-AChR did not lose receptors or develop clinical disease (Fig. 8.1). The early parts of

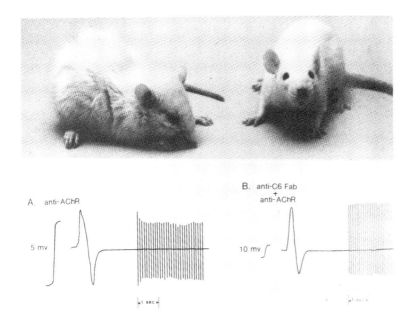

*Figure 8.1* Effect of C6 depletion on experimental myasthenia gravis (EAMG).
EAMG induced in mice by injection of antiacetylcholine receptor (anti-AChR) with or without Fab fragment of anti-C6. *Top*: animal on left, anti-AChR alone; on right, anti-AChR plus anti-C6. *Bottom*: markedly reduced electromyographic response in anti-AChR treated animal (left) as compared to relatively normal response in animal treated with anti-AChR plus anti-C6. From Biesecker and Gomez, *J. Immunol.* **142**, 2654–2659 (1989), with permission.

the pathway and all the inflammatory cell recruiting elements were intact in these animals, suggesting that the ability to form the membrane attack complex (MAC) is critical for pathology.

### 8.2.2 Complement and human myasthenia gravis

Changes at the motor endplate in MG resemble those seen in the experimental disease, although cellular infiltration is minimal or absent. The postsynaptic membrane is smooth and contains reduced numbers of AChRs. Antibody and complement components C3 and C9 (indicative of MAC formation) are present on the membrane, and

C9 is also found on fragments of membrane in the synaptic space (Fig. 8.2). The presence of MAC components on the postsynaptic membrane has led investigators to suggest that receptor loss occurs subsequent to 'microlysis', focal destruction by the MAC resulting in loss of membrane together with receptors. Perhaps a more likely explanation, in the light of our current knowledge of nucleated cell resistance to MAC killing, is that receptors are lost together with MACs during cell recovery either by endocytosis or exocytosis (see Section 1.3.3.4). The MAC-rich 'fragments' identified in the synaptic cleft may therefore represent membrane vesicles shed during recovery.

The levels of complement components or activation products in the sera of individuals with MG have not been examined to date. In view of the histological evidence presented above, it is probable that such studies will reveal ongoing classical-pathway activation in patients with active disease.

## 8.3 COMPLEMENT IN MULTIPLE SCLEROSIS

Multiple sclerosis (MS) is a chronic inflammatory demyelinating disease of unknown aetiology and variable clinical course. It is one of the commonest neurological diseases, particularly in temperate climates where the prevalence may exceed 1 in 1000. As might be expected for a common and crippling disease the cause of MS has been pursued aggressively, and many factors have been implicated. Viral, genetic, immunological, dietary and many other potential causes have been explored but it is likely that no single factor is entirely responsible for pathogenesis.

Currently, two contrasting but not mutually exclusive hypotheses predominate, the first being that MS is an autoimmune disease and the second that it is caused by a persistent virus infection of the central nervous system (CNS). Evidence for an involvement of the immune system in MS has been provided by the demonstration of increased levels of immunoglobulin, immune complexes and T and B lymphocytes in the brain and cerebrospinal fluid (CSF). Immunoglobulin in the CSF can be shown by electrophoresis to be composed of a limited number of discrete isotypes, each the product of a B-cell clone (oligoclonal response). Most of these clonal immunoglobulins do not recognize specific antigens but occasionally antibodies against CNS components are found.

Complement in Multiple Sclerosis   145

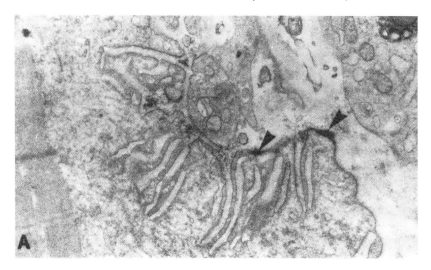

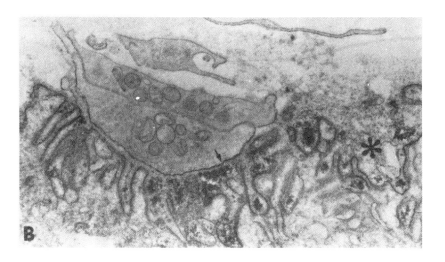

*Figure 8.2* Terminal complement deposition in myasthenia gravis (MG).
Complement component C9 localised in MG muscle by immunoperoxidase staining.
(A, B) Polyclonal antibody localizes C9 to endplate regions (arrowed in (A)).
Magnification × 1600. From Sahashi *et al.*, *J. Neuropathol. Exp. Neurol.* **39**, 160–172
(1980), with permission.

There is abundant evidence implicating cell mediated immunity in the pathogenesis of MS and this is described in several reviews listed at the end of this chapter. Despite the aforementioned immunoglobulin abnormalities, the involvement of humoral immunity in MS has attracted much less attention. The role of complement in demyelination has been examined using explants of neural tissue *in vitro*, in animal models and recently in the human disease. These studies are described in the following sections.

### 8.3.1 Complement and demyelination *in vitro*

It was demonstrated over 25 years ago that serum and/or CSF from some patients with MS caused demyelination of myelinated cultures of rat neural tissue. The morphology of demyelination in this system closely resembles that seen in the CNS of patients with MS. Serum from animals with experimental allergic encephalomyelitis, the principal model for MS, also causes demyelination *in vitro*. Demyelinating activity was shown to require IgG (or IgM) antibody and a heat-labile serum component, suggesting that it is mediated by antimyelin antibody activating complement via the classical pathway. Antibody-independent activation of complement by myelin itself has also been demonstrated *in vitro*; thus antibody may not be an essential requirement for demyelination. Involvement of complement in demyelination in these model systems has been confirmed using sera depleted of complement components. Antimyelin antibody and whole serum cause demyelination *in vitro* whereas antibody and C8-depleted serum do not, implicating complement and specifically the MAC.

In the CNS myelin is synthesized by oligodendrocytes. It has recently been shown that these cells activate homologous complement *in vitro* via the classical pathway in the absence of antibody, and are extremely susceptible to damage by the homologous MAC. It is therefore possible that exposure of neural tissue to high levels of complement *in vivo*, perhaps as a result of blood–brain barrier breakdown, specifically damages oligodendrocytes, thus causing demyelination.

## 8.3.2 Complement and animal models of multiple sclerosis

Experimental allergic encephalomyelitis (EAE) is induced in experimental animals by immunization with CNS tissue or purified CNS antigens in Freund's complete adjuvant. About 10 days after immunization, susceptible animals develop an acute neurological disease characterized by progressive weakness and weight loss which can lead to death. Surviving animals recover completely over the course of about a week and, in most variants of the disease, there is no recurrence of symptoms. In the CNS perivascular lymphocytic infiltration is the predominant feature and demyelination is minimal or absent, particularly when induced by purified CNS antigens. Despite these obvious differences from MS, which is a chronic demyelinating disease, EAE has been much studied as a model for the human disease. Various strategies have been employed to develop forms of EAE which more closely resemble MS. Demyelination has been produced by injection of antibodies against CNS antigens at the onset of clinical symptoms, and relapsing disease has been induced in some strains of guinea pigs.

EAE has long been considered a T-cell-mediated disease, based on the observation that disease can be transferred from a diseased animal to a naive recipient by transfusion of T cells. Despite this finding, evidence that complement is required for the full expression of clinical disease has been described. Decomplementation of animals by treatment with CVF ameliorates clinical disease induced actively (immunization with CNS antigens) or passively (T cell transfer), particularly when the antigenic or T-cell challenge is small (Fig. 8.3). Granular deposition of C9 — indicative of MAC formation — is detectable in the CNS in EAE, particularly in areas of active demyelination, suggesting that in the model disease, as demonstrated *in vitro*, MAC formation is involved in myelin damage.

Recently, interest has focussed on a second experimental disease as a model for MS. It was demonstrated over 50 years ago that infection of mice with Theiler's virus induced encephalomyelitis. The disease is accompanied by demyelination and its similarity to MS has been noted, particularly by those favouring a viral aetiology for the human disease. Unlike EAE, which is clearly an autoimmune disease, there is no evidence for autoimmunity in Theiler's virus encephalomyelitis, and no data exists to implicate complement in demyelination in this disease. Which of these experimental diseases provides the more appropriate model for human MS remains to be ascertained.

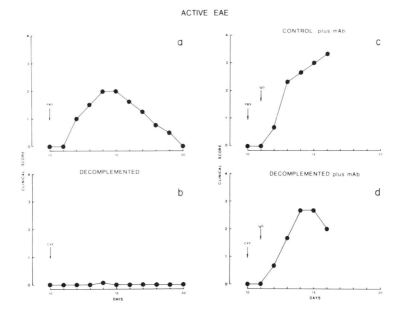

*Figure 8.3* Effect of decomplementation on experimental allergic encephalomyelitis (EAE).
Lewis rats were inoculated with myelin basic protein in adjuvant on day 0 and divided into four groups. Ten days later, half the animals (groups b and d) were decomplemented using CVF. The following day groups c (normal complement) and d (decomplemented) were injected with a demyelinating antibody. Animals were scored daily for clinical disease on a scale of 0 (no disease) to 4 (moribund or dead). Groups a and b demonstrate the ablation of the nondemyelinating disease by decomplementation. Groups c and d show exacerbation of disease by antibody and its amelioration by decomplementation. From Morgan, *Complement Inflamm.* **6**, 104–111 (1989), with permission.

### 8.3.3 Complement in human multiple sclerosis

As noted above, immunoglobulins, some of which may be complement-fixing antibodies, and immune complexes are found in increased amounts in the CSF and brain tissue of individuals with MS. The potential for complement activation in the CNS is thus clearly present. Complement components and activation complexes have been measured in the CSF in MS with rather variable results. Levels of C2 and C3 are normal and C4 is slightly reduced in comparison to control CSF. Low levels of C9 have been found in some patients and the terminal complement complex is detectable, suggesting terminal complement activation in the CNS. Using antibodies specific for the complex the MAC has been identified in

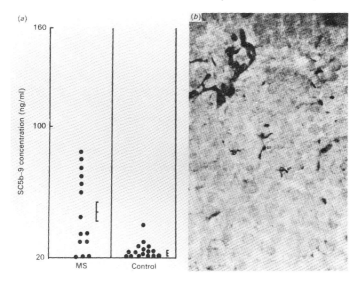

*Figure 8.4* Cerebrospinal fluid and tissue terminal complement complexes (TCCs) in multiple sclerosis.

(*a*) Concentrations of TCCs in the cerebrospinal fluid of multiple sclerosis patients compared with those in control individuals. Bars represent mean plus or minus standard error for each group. (*b*) A plaque from the brain of a patient with multiple sclerosis stained with TCC-specific antibodies. Granular staining is present in capillaries (arrowed). From Morgan, *Biochem. J.* **264**, 1–14 (1989), with permission.

the brain. The MAC is present as granular deposits in the walls of small blood vessels both in plaques and in grossly normal white matter, but is not detectable by light microscopy outside blood vessels (Fig. 8.4).

The mechanism(s) of complement activation and MAC formation within the CNS and the contribution these factors make to the overall pathogenesis of MS remain to be established. However, the evidence from *in vitro* and model systems suggests that complement may contribute substantially to oligodendrocyte damage and myelin breakdown in the human disease. The data implicating complement in demyelination *in vitro* and in animal and human disease are summarized in Table 8.1.

Table 8.1 Complement in demyelination.

| Source | Evidence |
| --- | --- |
| In vitro | MS/EAE serum causes demyelination in organ culture (IgG and complement required); antibody-independent activation of complement by myelin (demyelination requires MAC); oligodendrocytes activate homologous complement |
| Animal model (EAE) | Decomplementation with CVF ameliorates; C9 deposition in the CNS in areas of demyelination |
| Human disease (MS) | CSF C4 and C9 levels low and TCCs detectable; membrane fragments bearing MACs in CSF; MAC deposition in brain |

MS, multiple sclerosis; EAE, experimental allergic encephalomyelitis; CSF, cerebrospinal fluid; MAC, membrane attack complex; TCC, terminal complement complex.

## 8.4 COMPLEMENT IN OTHER NEUROLOGICAL DISEASES

Measurement of complement components or activation products in the CSF and in the brain have implicated complement in a number of other inflammatory diseases of the nervous system. The evidence for a role of complement in the neurological syndrome associated with systemic lupus erythematosus were described in Section 6.4.4. Complement activation products have also been identified in the CSF in subacute sclerosing panencephalomyelitis (SSPE) and in Sjogren's syndrome with CNS involvement. It is likely that complement activation in all three of these diseases occurs subsequent to immune complex formation in the CNS.

In SSPE the underlying aetiology is a chronic infection of the CNS with measles virus. Extremely high titres of antiviral antibodies are found in the CSF and complement-activating immune complexes are formed. In the early stages of infection complement-mediated lysis of infected cells occurs in the presence of antiviral antibody, thus limiting disease progression, albeit at a cost in terms of neural cell loss (Section 5.2). As a consequence of surface antigen modulation and perhaps also of CSF complement depletion, a proportion of infected cells escape lysis, establishing a persistent viral infection in the CNS.

Guillain–Barré syndrome is characterized by the acute or subacute onset of generalized polyneuropathy. Motor, sensory and cranial nerves may all be involved, although the clinical presentation is very variable. The disease may follow a viral infection or may arise spontaneously. Death may occur due to respiratory paralysis, but most individuals recover over the course of weeks or months and the disease rarely recurs. Serum from patients contains an antibody against Schwann cells which, in the presence of complement, causes demyelination of myelinated nerve cultures *in vitro*. Despite this observation, relatively little is known about the role of complement in the pathogenesis of either the human disease or its animal model, experimental allergic neuritis. Elevated levels of terminal complement complexes have been found in the CSF in Guillain–Barré syndrome, providing evidence of complement activation in the CNS, although the relevance of this finding to the pathogenesis of a disease which affects primarily the peripheral nervous system is unclear.

Alzheimer's disease is a chronic degenerative disease of the CNS characterized clinically by progressive dementia and pathologically by diffuse cerebral atrophy. The histological features include senile plaques, neurofibrillary tangles, dystrophic neurites and amyloid formation. Although many factors have been implicated the pathogenesis of the disease remains uncertain. Complement components, including C1, C3 and C4, have been identified in senile plaques and amyloid, and the terminal complement complex (MAC) has recently been localized in neurofibrillary tangles and dystrophic neurites. Alternative-pathway components are not found in these regions, implying that activation occurs via the classical pathway. Although there is no evidence that complement activation is a primary factor in the pathogenesis of this disease, its contribution to neurone loss may be of significance and certainly merits further investigation. The evidence for an involvement of complement in these other neurological diseases is summarized in Table 8.2.

## 8.5 COMPLEMENT AND DISEASES OF MUSCLE

The term *polymyositis* encompasses a group of inflammatory disorders of muscle which share an underlying autoimmune aetiology. Inflammation may be restricted to muscle (chronic polymyositis) or may also involve the skin (dermatomyositis), and in either case may be an isolated finding or may occur in association with other autoimmune diseases, particularly systemic lupus erythematosus and scleroderma. In the early stages affected muscles become tender, swollen and weak. Chronic changes include progressive wasting and weakness. Muscle biopsy reveals cellular

Table 8.2 Complement in other neurological diseases.

| Disease | Evidence |
| --- | --- |
| Systemic lupus erythematosus (cerebral lupus) | Presence of TCCs and decreased C4 levels in CSF |
| Sjorgren's syndrome (with CNS involvement) | Presence of TCCs in CSF |
| Subacute sclerosing panencephalitis | Complement activating immune complexes and complement depletion in CSF; complement-mediated neuronal loss |
| Guillain–Barré syndrome | Complement fixing anti-Schwann cell antibody causes demyelination *in vitro*; TCCs in CSF |
| Alzheimer's syndrome | C3, C4, C1 and MAC all localized in plaques |
| Chronic relapsing polyneuropathy | C3 deposits in intraneural blood vessels |

CSF, cerebrospinal fluid; TCC, terminal complement complex; MAC, membrane attack complex.

infiltration and fragmentation of muscle fibres. In the majority of patients antibodies to myoglobin are present in the circulation, but whether these are of primary significance or merely represent a secondary response to muscle cell lysis is unclear.

Deposition of complement has been demonstrated in diseased muscle in polymyositis. Early studies showed dense deposits of C3 and C9 in association with necrotic fibres. Although a role for complement in fibre damage was suggested in these studies, it was not possible to exclude the possibility that complement activation occurred merely as a secondary response to necrotic tissue. More recently, C9 (and by inference the MAC) has been localized on the surfaces of histologically normal fibres in polymyositis, directly implicating complement in fibre damage (Fig. 8.5).

Although childhood dermatomyositis is clinically similar to polymyositis, its aetiology appears to be different. Vascular abnormalities are detectable in skeletal muscle and other organs and it has been suggested that the disease is the result of a widespread small-vessel angiopathy. Heavy deposits of the MAC have been demonstrated not only on necrotic muscle fibres but also in the intramuscular small vessels of patients with this disease, and it has been suggested that MAC-mediated vessel injury is the primary pathogenic factor in this condition.

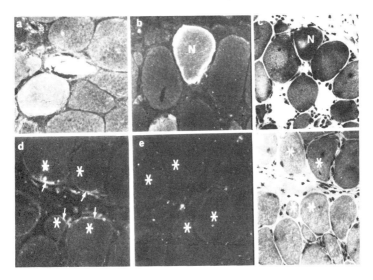

*Figure 8.5* Localization of complement component C9 in myositis.
Sections of muscle from a patient with myositis. (*a, b, d, e*) Double antibody immunofluorescence staining using anti-C9 monoclonal antibody (MC47) as first antibody (all × 255): (*a*) C9 in a necrotic fibre; (*b*) C9 localized to the periphery of a large, prenecrotic fibre (N); (*c*) serial section of (*b*) stained with haemotoxylin and eosin showing patchy staining in fibre N (× 170); (*d*) C9 in discrete patches (arrowed) on the surface of four fibres; (*e*) serial section of (*d*) using C9-saturated antibody as a control; (*f*) serial section of (*d*) stained with haemotoxylin and eosin showing normal appearance of the same fibres (× 170). From Morgan *et al.*, *Immunology* **52**, 181–188 (1984), with permission.

The muscular dystrophies are a group of inherited disorders characterized by progressive degeneration of certain muscle groups. The aetiology of muscle damage in these conditions was until very recently completely unknown. The gene for the commonest form of muscular dystrophy, the X-linked Duchenne dystrophy (DMD), has now been isolated and absence of a sarcolemmal protein, dystrophin, in DMD has been implicated in pathogenesis. Although the mechanisms of pathogenesis in DMD remain unknown, its association with absence of a sarcolemmal protein suggests an underlying membrane defect. Complement component C9 (indicative of MAC formation) has been located in muscle from individuals with DMD, the distribution being similar to that described in polymyositis. The relevance of this finding to muscle damage in this condition remains to be determined.

## 8.6 COMPLEMENT IN NEUROLOGICAL AND MUSCULAR DISEASES

From the above account it is clear that evidence has been produced suggestive of a role of complement in a diverse group of neurological and muscular diseases. In every case other potentially pathogenic candidates exist and complement must always be considered as just one component in a complex web of interacting factors. However, the complement system may be more amenable to therapeutic intervention than some of these other factors, and therefore its role and relative importance in these diseases should be clarified.

## 8.7 FURTHER READING

*Myasthenia gravis*

Newsom-Davis, J. and Vincent, A. (1982). Myasthenia gravis. In: Lachmann, P. J. and Peters, D. K. (eds), *Clinical Aspects of Immunology*. Blackwell, Oxford, pp. 1011–1068.

Lennon, V. A., Seybold, M. E., Lindstrom, J. M., Cochrane, C. and Ulevitch, R. (1978). Role of complement in the pathogenesis of experimental autoimmune myasthenia gravis. *J. Exp. Med.* **147**, 973–983.

Sahashi, K., Engel, A. G., Lambert, E. H. and Howard, F. M. (1980). Ultrastructural localisation of the terminal and lytic ninth complement component (C9) at the end plate in myasthenia gravis. *J. Neuropathol. Exp. Neurol.* **39**, 160–172.

Biesecker, G. and Gomez, C. M. (1989). Inhibition of acute passive transfer experimental autoimmune myasthenia gravis with Fab antibody to complement C6. *J. Immunol.* **142**, 2654–2659.

*Multiple sclerosis*

Sayetta, R. B. (1986). Theories of the aetiology of multiple sclerosis: a critical review. *J. Clin. Lab. Immunol.* **21**, 55–70.

Turner, A., Cuzner, M. L., Davison, A. N. and Rudge, P. (1980). On the role of sensitised T-lymphocytes in the pathogenesis of multiple sclerosis. *J. Neurol. Neurosurg. Psychiatr.* **43**, 305–309.

Arnason, B. G. W. (1983). Immunology of multiple sclerosis. In: Franklin, E. C. (ed.), *Clinical Immunology Update*. Elsevier Biomedical, New York, pp. 235–259.

Caspary, E. A. (1984). Humoral factors involved in immune processes in multiple sclerosis and allergic encephalomyelitis. *Br. Med. Bull.* **33**, 50–53.

Liu, W. T., Vanguri, P. and Shin, M. L. (1983). Studies on demyelination *in vitro*: the requirement of membrane attack components of the complement system. *J. Immunol.* **131**, 778–782.

Compston, D. A. S., Morgan, B. P., Campbell, A. K., Wilkins, P., Cole, G., Thomas, N. D. and Jasani, B. (1989). Immunocytochemical localization of the terminal complement complex in multiple sclerosis. *Neuropathol. Appl. Neurobiol.* **15**, 307–316.

*Others*

Sanders, M. E., Alexander, E. L., Koski, C. L., Frank, M. M. and Joiner, K. A. (1987). Detection of activated terminal complement (C5b–9) in cerebrospinal fluid from patients with central nervous system involvement of primary Sjogren's syndrome or systemic lupus erythematosus. *J. Immunol.* **138**, 2095–2099.

Morgan, B. P., Sewry, C. A., Siddle, K., Luzio, J. P. and Campbell, A. K. (1984). Immunolocalisation of complement component C9 on necrotic and non-necrotic muscle fibres in myositis using monoclonal antibodies. *Immunology* **52**, 181–187.

Kissel, J. T., Mendel, J. R. and Rammohan, K. W. (1986). Microvascular deposition of complement membrane attack complex in dermatomyositis. *N. Engl. J. Med.* **314**, 329–334.

McGeer, P. L., Akiyama, H., Itagaki, S. and McGeer, E. G. (1989). Activation of the classical complement pathway in brain tissue of Alzheimer patients. *Neurosci. Lett.* **107**, 341–346.

CHAPTER NINE
# Complement and Dermatological Diseases

## 9.1 INTRODUCTION

Diseases of the skin are particularly amenable to investigation because it is relatively easy to obtain portions of the affected tissue for biochemical, immunological and histological testing. Despite this advantage, the aetiology of many skin diseases is poorly understood. The immune system has been implicated in a variety of dermatological diseases, often because of their association with other diseases of autoimmune aetiology or with specific HLA allotypes. Both cell-mediated and humoral mechanisms have been demonstrated or postulated in skin diseases. The relevance of complement has recently attracted attention in bullous (or blistering) conditions, in various forms of urticaria and angioedema and in vasculitic skin diseases. Patients with complement deficiencies or abnormalities of control proteins frequently present with skin pathology. The evidence for an involvement of complement in the pathogenesis of these groups of diseases is presented in this chapter.

## 9.2 COMPLEMENT AND BULLOUS DISEASES

Several skin diseases are characterized by blistering, the distribution and properties of the blisters varying among the different conditions. Included in this group are pemphigus vulgaris, bullous pemphigoid, herpes gestationis and dermatitis herpetiformis. In these diseases autoimmune mechanisms, initiated primarily by autoantibodies, have been implicated. The role of complement has been examined in each disease and the conclusions of these studies are presented below and summarized in Table 9.1.

## 9.2.1 Complement in pemphigus vulgaris

Pemphigus vulgaris (PV) is a chronic disease characterized by flaccid blisters appearing on otherwise normal skin and on mucous membranes. The skin surrounding the lesions, though superficially normal, is highly sensitive to shearing forces, and pressure on the perilesional skin can greatly enlarge the blister, demonstrating the true extent of pathology. The blisters are intraepidermal and are caused by a loss of cohesion between individual epidermal cells — *acantholysis*.

Antibodies directed against antigens located in the intracellular substance of the epidermis and perhaps on the epidermal cells themselves are present in the serum of patients with PV. Purified PV immunoglobulin causes acantholysis when incubated with cultured explants of normal skin. Evidence has been produced that this is the result of antibody-stimulated release of proteases from epidermal cells which digest the intercellular substance. Antibody-induced acantholysis of skin explants is relatively inefficient, requiring high concentrations of immunoglobulin. In the presence of complement, however, acantholysis *in vitro* is greatly enhanced, and activated complement components are present in the intercellular substance and are deposited together with the MAC on epidermal cells.

*In vivo*, an involvement of complement is suggested by the demonstration of complement consumption and activation products — including chemotactic factors — in blister fluid. The fluid in suction blisters produced on skin in normal individuals contains complement levels close to those in serum, and very low levels of activation products, implying that activation in PV is disease-specific. Immunohistology of affected skin in PV reveals deposition of components of both the classical and alternative pathways in lesions and surrounding 'normal' skin in close proximity to immunoglobulin. Recently, terminal components and the MAC have been identified. Unlike the earlier components, the MAC appears to be restricted to lesions (Fig. 9.1). A direct toxic effect of the MAC on epidermal cells has been postulated to be of major pathogenic importance in PV.

## Complement and Dermatological Diseases

Table 9.1 Complement in bullous diseases.

| Disease | Deposits | Location | Other evidence |
|---|---|---|---|
| Pemphigus vulgaris | IgG, C1, C3, C4, FB, FH, P, MAC | ICS | Complement activation in blister fluid |
| Bullous pemphigoid | IgG, C1, C3, C3d, FB, P, C5, MAC | EBM | Complement activation in blister fluid |
| Dermatitis herpetiformis | IgA, C3, FB, P, MAC | Dermal papillae | — |
| Herpes gestationis | IgG, C3, FB, P, MAC | EBM | Hypocomplementaemia in acute phase |
| Erythema multiforme | IgM, C3 | BV | — |
| Epidermolysis bullosa acquisita | IgG, IgA, C3, C4, C3d, P, C5 | EBM | — |
| Porphyria cutanea tarda | C3, IgG | BV | — |

FB, FH, Factors B and H; P, properdin; MAC, membrane attack complex; ICS, intercellular substance; EBM, epidermal basement membrane; BV, dermal blood vessels.

### 9.2.2 Complement in bullous pemphigoid

Bullous pemphigoid (BP) is a generalized blistering disorder characterized by rigid, subepidermal blisters with inflamed bases. Immunohistology reveals deposition of immunoglobulin and C3 at the dermal–epidermal junction in association with the basement membrane. Deposition of C3 in these areas is an important diagnostic criterion in BP, being present in virtually all cases, unlike antibody which is not detectable by standard techniques in about 20%. More than 80% of patients with BP have complement fixing antibasement membrane antibody in their serum. These findings, together with the demonstration of complement consumption and activation products in blister fluid (as described above for PV), have firmly implicated complement in pathogenesis. However, the exact mechanisms of complement activation and its contribution to pathogenesis remain unclear.

Complement activation at the dermal–epidermal junction releases chemotactic and anaphylactic peptides which attract neutrophils and

*Figure 9.1* Complement in pemphigus vulgaris and bullous pemphigoid.
Complement C3 and the MAC localized using specific antibodies in perilesional skin of patients with pemphigus vulgaris (PV) and bullous pemphigoid (BP). (*A*, *B*) Staining for C3 and MAC respectively in PV. Staining predominantly intercellular (× 160). (*C*, *D*) Staining for C3 and MAC respectively in BP. Dense linear staining of basement membrane (× 160). (*A*) and (*B*) from Kawana *et al.*, *J. Invest. Dermatol.* **92**, 588–592 (1989); (*C*) from Jordon *et al.*, *J. Invest. Dermatol.* **85**, 72s–78s (1985); (*D*) from Dahl *et al.*, *J. Invest. Dermatol.* **82**, 132–135 (1984), all with permission.

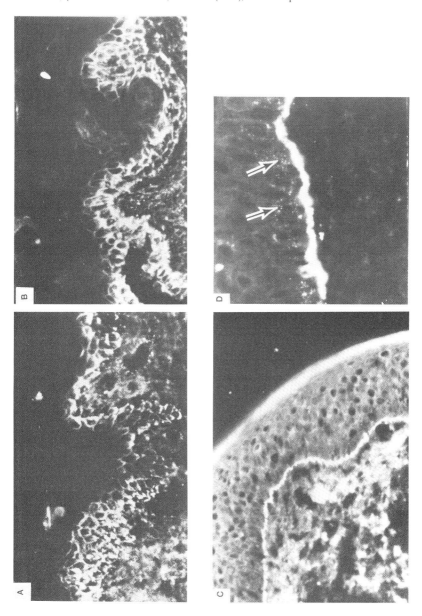

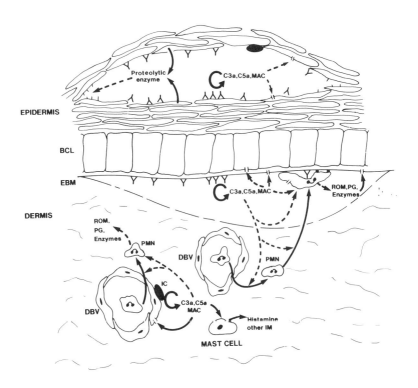

*Figure 9.2* Schematic representation of complement-mediated skin damage. The diagram illustrates the role of complement in three skin diseases. In pemphigus vulgaris (PV), antibodies against the epidermal cells and the intracellular substance directly cause the release of enzymes from cells and, in association with antigen, activate complement. Acantholysis results from a combination of these factors. In bullous pemphigoid (BP), antibasement membrane antibodies in association with antigen activate complement. Released chemotactic factors attract neutrophils (PMN) to the dermal–epidermal junction where they bind to the basement membrane and are stimulated to release toxic factors which disrupt the junction. The MAC may also damage the basement membrane and the basal epidermal cells directly. In cutaneous vasculitis, immune complexes form or are deposited in dermal blood vessels where they activate complement. C3a and C5a attract neutrophils into the tissues and activate them and mast cells to release inflammatory mediators. The MAC may damage endothelial cells directly, exacerbating vessel destruction. BCL, basal cell layer; EBM, epidermal basement membrane; DBV, dermal blood vessel; PMN, neutrophil; ROM, reactive oxygen metabolite; PG, prostaglandin; IM, inflammatory mediator.

other inflammatory cells to the site, and stimulate the release of proteolytic enzymes from neutrophils. Neutrophil enzymes have been implicated in separation and blister formation. In some individuals with BP the lesions contain few inflammatory cells, and in these cases neutrophil-mediated damage cannot be the major factor. An alternative possibility is that complement damages the dermal–epidermal junction directly. Complement components, including the MAC, are present in large amounts in this region (Fig. 9.1) and the MAC may itself disrupt the basement membrane or cause the release of damaging factors from adjacent cells (Fig. 9.2).

### 9.2.3 Complement in dermatitis herpetiformis

Dermatitis herpetiformis (DH) is a chronic bullous disease characterized by small, tense, subepidermal blisters on an erythematous base with intense itching of affected areas. The skin pathology is accompanied by small-bowel changes which resemble closely those seen in coeliac disease, but malabsorption is rare in DH. Both the skin and gut changes respond to removal of gluten from the diet, providing further evidence for a relationship to coeliac disease.

Immunofluorescent examination of biopsies from DH patients reveals granular or linear deposits of IgA around the lesion and also in skin remote from lesions. C3, Factor B and properdin are also found around the lesion, but C4 and C1 are not usually detected, suggesting that complement activation occurs in this disease predominantly via the alternative pathway. The MAC has also been identified in and around lesions and, as with PV and BP, a pathogenic role for this complex has been proposed. However, the symptoms of DH often respond dramatically to treatment with sulphone, a drug which has no detectable effect on complement activation, and low-grade complement deposition in skin continues despite successful treatment. These findings imply that additional noncomplement factors are involved in the pathogenesis of DH.

### 9.2.4 Complement in herpes gestationis

Herpes gestationis (HG) is a rare, self-limiting blistering disease which appears during or soon after pregnancy. The skin lesions are rather variable but commonly are large, tense blisters covering much of the body. Histologically the disease is characterized by destruction of the basal cell layer of the epidermis. Immunofluorescence reveals heavy deposition of C3, and lighter deposits of properdin and Factor B in the region of the basement membrane, suggesting alternative-pathway activation. Using standard histochemical techniques immunoglobulin is detected in the tissues in less than one-half the cases, but low levels of complement fixing antibasement membrane antibody activity can be detected in the serum of most HG patients.

Despite the heavy and widespread deposition of C3, the serum complement levels are usually normal in HG. However, during the acute phase of lesion eruption, significant hypocomplementaemia and evidence of activation of both the classical and alternative pathways have been reported.

### 9.2.5 Complement in the porphyrias

The porphyrias are a group of diseases each of which is caused by a specific enzyme defect in the pathway of haem biosynthesis. Haem precursors accumulate in the serum and tissues. In several of these diseases the precursors (porphyrins) which accumulate cause skin reactions ranging from mild erythema to severe blistering and scarring in areas exposed to sunlight. Deposition of complement (C3) and immunoglobulin around blood vessels and at the dermal–epidermal junction has been reported in perilesional and sun-exposed skin in all the forms of porphyria associated with photosensitivity. Further, irradiation of nonlesional skin causes capillary endothelial cell lysis, mast cell degranulation and neutrophil accumulation in the dermis, all of which may be accounted for by complement activation.

*In vitro*, activation of complement occurs in normal serum spiked with porphyrins and irradiated with light of the appropriate wavelength (400–410 nm), although the molecular mechanisms by which activation occurs are unknown. It has been suggested that photoactivation of complement may be responsible for the skin lesions not only in the porphyrias but also in phototoxic reactions to drugs. Evidence for this has been provided by animal studies. For example, chlorpromazine-induced phototoxicity in guinea pigs is accompanied by the appearance of complement activation products in the serum, and clinical symptoms are markedly ameliorated by prior decomplementation of the animals using CVF.

Even in normal individuals small amounts of complement deposition at the dermal–epidermal junction are detectable in areas of skin exposed to sunlight, implying that photoactivation of complement occurs even in the absence of abnormal phototoxic molecules, and may be a factor in the causation of sunburn.

## 9.3 COMPLEMENT AND URTICARIA

Urticaria and angioedema are characterized by transient, localized areas of oedema involving the dermis and/or the subcutaneous tissues. In urticaria the oedema involves predominantly the superficial parts of the dermis, whereas in angioedema it involves mainly the subcutaneous tissue. The separation of these two conditions is rather artificial and both can occur together. In the majority of individuals the initiating stimulus for urticaria is not known. In a minority the skin reaction follows exposure to a known allergen or physical stimulus. Most cases, even of physical urticaria or angioedema, are due to Type I anaphylactic reactions mediated by IgE antibody.

Angioedema associated with congenital or acquired deficiency of C1 inhibitor is described in Section 4.3.5. The evidence for complement involvement in other forms of urticaria and angioedema is much more tenuous. Urticaria and angioedema may be the sole or major presenting feature of a systemic disease such as serum sickness or systemic lupus erythematosus, and in these instances may be associated with marked hypocomplementaemia. Whether immune complex deposition and complement activation in the skin is responsible for the symptoms in these individuals is unclear. In the majority of cases of urticaria and angioedema uncomplicated by systemic disease or by vasculitis (see below), there is no evidence for complement activation or deposition in the skin.

## 9.4 COMPLEMENT IN CUTANEOUS VASCULITIC SYNDROMES

Vasculitis is characterized by inflammation of blood vessels. In the skin the cutaneous venules are involved, producing urticarial and/or purpuric erythematous lesions. Vasculitis is rarely restricted to the skin but involvement of internal organs is often not clinically obvious.

The presence of immunoglobulin in the vessel walls of lesional

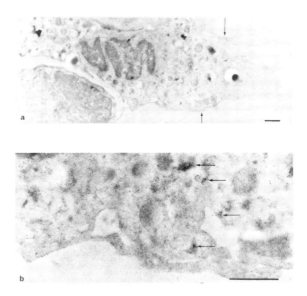

*Figure 9.3* MAC in cutaneous vasculitis.
Electron micrographs of a vessel wall in immune complex vasculitis of the skin. (*a*) Neutrophil penetrating the endothelial cell wall (arrowed) (× 9000). (*b*). Detail of (*a*) showing deposits of MAC (immunogold labelled, arrowed) (× 30 000). The bar in each micrograph is 1 μm. From Boom *et al.*, *J. Invest. Dermatol.* **93**, 68s–72s (1989), with permission.

skin in vasculitis was first noted over 30 years ago. Complement C3 co-localizes with immunoglobulin in a variety of different forms of vasculitis, including necrotizing (leucocytoclastic) vasculitis. More recently, activation products, including fragments of C3 and C4, and the MAC, have been demonstrated in lesional skin in most individuals with vasculitis. The MAC is present on the surface of endothelial cells of the dermal vessels and on infiltrating neutrophils, and appears to be involved directly in endothelial cell damage or destruction (Fig. 9.3). Damage to endothelial cells has been assumed to be due to the release of lysosomal enzymes and other active products from infiltrating neutrophils. Formation of nonlethal amounts of the MAC on these cells may be the stimulus for release of these inflammatory mediators, contributing to endothelial cell damage and enhancing local inflammation (see Section 2.2.5 and Fig. 9.2).

## 9.5 SKIN DISEASE IN COMPLEMENT DEFICIENCY STATES

The various complement deficiencies and their clinical consequences are detailed in Chapter 4. This section highlights those complement deficiencies which are associated with skin disease. The involvement of C1 inhibitor deficiency in angioedema is described in Section 4.3.5. Complement deficiencies are rare, and in all the skin disorders mentioned only a small percentage of cases are associated with deficiencies.

Skin disease is common among individuals deficient in classical pathway components. Most patients have either discoid (DLE) or systemic (SLE) lupus erythematosus. DLE is particularly frequent among individuals with deficiencies of C1q and C2. The clinical picture consists of chronic erythematous, scaling, discoid lesions usually on the face which eventually cause scarring. Symptoms are aggravated by exposure to sunlight and lesions are usually restricted to exposed areas. The disease is closely related to SLE but systemic symptoms are mild or absent.

The skin lesions in SLE are very variable. The commonest pattern is a blotchy erythematous eruption of the face and neck, but symptoms may range from a mild rash to marked skin loss and scarring. Biopsy of skin lesions reveals basal cell damage and immunoglobulin deposition. Deficiencies of C1q, C1r, C2, C4 and C3 are all associated with SLE, C2 deficiency being by far the most frequent. Absence of the controlling proteins Factor H and Factor I causes depletion of C3, and thus a secondary deficiency, and can present with SLE.

The hypocomplementaemic cutaneous vasculitis syndrome is another SLE-related skin disease associated with complete or partial deficiencies of complement components. The skin lesions in this disease are typically urticarial, purpuric and pruritic, and biopsy shows small-vessel inflammation and necrosis. Whether this syndrome truly represents a distinct clinical entity or is merely one part of the spectrum of complement-deficiency SLE is not clear.

The pathology of tissue damage in complement deficiency SLE is described in Section 6.4.5. Occasionally, individuals with deficiencies of terminal components present with SLE-like symptoms, often predominantly cutaneous. The pathological basis in these cases is unknown (Section 4.3.4).

Deficiency of the complement receptor $CR_3$ is associated with a typical dermatological appearance. These individuals are extremely susceptible to infections of the skin, which heal leaving paper-thin scars (Section 4.3.5.3).

Although not often present in individuals with primary complement deficiency, partial lipodystrophy is closely associated with the presence of an abnormal complement activator, the C3 nephritic factor (C3NeF), an IgG autoantibody which stabilizes the C3 convertase of the alternative pathway (Section 4.3.5.5). In this condition there is symmetrical loss of subcutaneous fat, usually from the face, arms and trunk. In most patients with partial lipodystrophy there is evidence of complement activation, with low serum levels of C3 but normal C4 and C2, implying alternative-pathway activation. Partial lipodystrophy is frequently associated with nephritis, but hypocomplementaemia is present even in the absence of overt renal disease. The pathological basis of partial lipodystrophy and the role, if any, of complement activation remain unknown. It has been speculated that complement deficiency secondary to activation might predispose individuals to infectious agents which are responsible for the loss of subcutaneous fat. The dermatological symptoms associated with primary or secondary complement deficiencies are summarized in Table 9.2.

## 9.6 COMPLEMENT AND SKIN DISEASE

The above account describes those skin diseases for which there is most evidence implicating complement in pathology. Complement components have been demonstrated in and around lesions in a

*Table 9.2* Dermatological diseases associated with congenital or acquired complement deficiencies.

| Disease | Deficiencies |
|---|---|
| Angioedema | Inherited or acquired deficiency of C1inh |
| Discoid lupus, cutaneous vasculitis syndrome, systemic lupus erythematosus | Congenital or acquired deficiencies of classical-pathway components: C2, C1, C4 or C3 |
| Partial lipodystrophy | Deficiency of C3 secondary to activation by C3NeF |
| Lichen planus | Occasionally associated with C4 deficiency |
| Xeroderma pigmentosum | Rarely associated with C8 deficiency |
| Recurrent cutaneous infections | Deficiency of $CR_3$ |

large number of other skin diseases, although the relevance to pathology in these other conditions has not yet been explored. The importance of complement activation in skin pathology may not even be limited to disease. It has been demonstrated that the stratum corneum is itself an activator of the alternative pathway of complement. It has been suggested that exposure of stratum corneum to serum following traumatic injury or rupture of acne comedones causes activation of complement which initiates or perpetuates inflammation.

The dermatological disorders in which complement has been localized or implicated are listed in Table 9.3. As noted earlier, it is likely that damage in most of these conditions is multifactorial. However, if complement does contribute to pathogenesis, specific inhibitors of complement activation (Chapter 12) might be of therapeutic benefit. Skin diseases might be particularly suitable for

*Table 9.3* Complement in dermatological diseases.

| Disease | Tissue complement | Systemic complement |
|---|---|---|
| Immune complex vasculitis | C3, MAC in walls of dermal vessels | Hypocomplementaemia common |
| Systemic lupus erythematosus | C3, C1, P, FB beneath EBM in lesions | Hypocomplementaemia common |
| Discoid lupus erythematosus | C3 beneath EBM in lesions | Hypocomplementaemia rare |
| Vitiligo | C3 in areas of active depigmentation | N/ND |
| Lichen planus | C3, C1, C9 on EBM and on 'ovoid bodies' | N/ND |
| Acne rosacea | C3 beneath EBM in lesions | N/ND |
| Acne vulgaris | C3 on EBM and in vessels in lesions | N/ND |
| Psoriasis | C1, C3, C4 in epidermis and dermal vessels | N/ND |
| Pityrias lichenoides | C3 beneath EBM and in dermal vessels | N/ND |

MAC, membrane attack complex; P, properdin; FB, Factor B; EBM, epidermal basement membrane; N/ND, normal or not tested.

Involvement of complement in the bullous diseases is summarized in Table 9.1. Data in this table in part from Rauterberg, in: Rother and Till (eds), *The Complement System*, Springer, Berlin, pp. 287–326 (1988).

*Complement and Dermatological Diseases*

this sort of therapeutic intervention. In the same way that topical steroids have relieved the symptoms of dermatitis with minimal systemic effects, so specific complement inhibitors applied topically might dampen down dermal activation without disturbing complement function elsewhere.

## 9.7 FURTHER READING

Boom, B. W., Mommaas, M., Daha, M. R. and Vermeer, B. J. (1989). Complement-mediated endothelial cell damage in immune complex vasculitis of the skin: ultrastructural localization of the membrane attack complex. *J. Invest. Dermatol.* **93**, 68s–72s.

Boonk, W. J., Nieboer, C. and Huijgens, P. C. (1986). Pathogenic studies in chronic urticaria. *Dermatologica* **173**, 264–270.

Gigli, I. (1982). Immunological aspects of skin disease. In: Lachmann, P. J. and Peters, D. K. (eds), *Clinical Aspects of Immunology.* Blackwell, Oxford, pp. 790–821.

Jordon, R. E. (1979). The complement system in pemphigus and bullous pemphigoid. In: Beutner, E. H., Chorzelski, T. P. and Bean, S. F. (eds), *Immunopathology of the Skin.* Wiley, New York, pp. 135–145.

Jordan, R. E., Kawana, S. and Fritz, K. A. (1985). Immunopathologic mechanisms in pemphigus and bullous pemphigoid. *J. Invest. Dermatol.* **85**, 72s–78s.

Kawana, S., Geoghegan, W. D., Jordan, R. E. and Nishiyama, S. (1989). Deposition of the membrane attack complex of complement in pemphigus vulgaris and pemphigus foliaceus skin. *J. Invest. Dermatol.* **92**, 588–592.

Lim, H. and Gigli, I. (1981). The role of complement in phototoxic reactions. *Springer Semin. Immunopathol.* **4**, 209–219.

Sontheimer, R. D. and Gilliam, J. N. (1981). Immunologically mediated epidermal cell injury. *Springer Semin. Immunopathol.* **4**, 1–15.

CHAPTER TEN

# Complement in Iatrogenic and Post-traumatic Syndromes

## 10.1 INTRODUCTION

Complement activation has been implicated in the pathogenesis of several important syndromes occurring as a result or a complication of medical treatments, or secondary to major trauma, including surgical trauma. These syndromes are often predictable and potentially avoidable. Measurement of complement activation may be of predictive value and may also be useful in monitoring response to therapy. Strategies aimed at preventing or limiting activation may be therapeutically helpful. This chapter describes these syndromes and the evidence implicating complement.

## 10.2 COMPLEMENT ACTIVATION DUE TO BIOINCOMPATIBILITY

A wide variety of materials can activate complement *in vitro*, usually via the alternative pathway. In several clinical situations these materials are placed in contact with biological fluids and the potential therefore exists for complement activation *in vivo*. On a numerical basis, the most important situation where complement activation due to bioincompatibility occurs is in renal haemodialysis.

### 10.2.1 Complement and haemodialysis

During haemodialysis blood is exposed to an extensive area of foreign material. A variety of materials are used for the dialysis membranes and these differ markedly in their ability to activate complement. The most frequently used dialysis membranes are made of cuprophane, a material composed of repetitive polysaccharide units, which structurally resembles bacterial cell walls and the chromatography matrix Sephadex. In view of the well-known propensity of Sephadex and of bacteria to activate complement via the alternative pathway, it is not surprising that complement activation is a common accompaniment of haemodialysis using this material. Complement activation is evidenced by increased plasma levels of the anaphylatoxins C3a and C5a, of the terminal complement complex (TCC) and of the alternative-pathway-specific C3b,BbP complex (Section 12.2). In contrast, no increase in serum levels of the classical-pathway-specific C1/C1inh complex has been detected, demonstrating that activation occurs exclusively via the alternative pathway. Several other materials have been used as dialysis membranes (Table 10.1). Cellulose acetate membranes activate complement but to a much smaller extent than cuprophane, and membranes made of synthetic polymers, such as polycarbonate, polysulfone, polyacrylonitrile and polymethylmethacrylate, cause minimal activation. Upon second or subsequent use cuprophane membranes cause much less activation than when new, suggesting that the alternative-pathway activating sites are blocked during first exposure to blood. The degree of decrease in activation appears to be dependent on the method chosen for membrane sterilization (Table 10.1).

The clinical consequences of complement activation during dialysis may be serious. Large amounts of highly active products are released which will have both acute and long-term effects. Complement activation products may cause acute pulmonary inflammation directly, or may cause injury indirectly by stimulating the sequestration of neutrophils in the lung. A transient decrease in the numbers of circulating leucocytes is evident in most patients undergoing dialysis (particularly using a complement-activating membrane), and it is now clear that this leucopenia is the result of deposition of cells in the lung. During passage through the dialyser neutrophils and monocytes become coated with complement fragments, particularly C5a and C5adesArg, which cause activation. These activated cells aggregate and become deposited in the microvasculature of the lung where, by releasing enzymes and other

Table 10.1 Complement activation by dialysis membranes.

| Membrane | Degree of activation | Comments |
|---|---|---|
| Cuprophane (new) | ++++ | Cheap, simple to use |
| Cuprophane (re-used, Formalin sterilized) | + | Easiest strategy to minimize C activation |
| Cuprophane (re-used, Na$_2$ClO$_3$ sterilized) | +++ | |
| Cellulose acetate | + | |
| Polyacrylonitrile | +/− | Expensive, may require special equipment; bind C3a, C5a, and other active molecules; may reduce short- and long-term morbidity |
| Polyphenolymethylmethacrylate | +/− | |
| Polysulfone | +/− | |
| Polycarbonate | +/− | |

toxic molecules, they cause tissue damage. Acute pulmonary symptoms occur only rarely, although a transient decrease in lung function can be detected during dialysis in most patients. It has been suggested that the pulmonary fibrosis and calcinosis which occur in up to 60% of patients on long-term dialysis are due to repeated complement- or neutrophil-induced lung injury. Endothelial damage by activated neutrophils has also been proposed to contribute to the accelerated atheroma associated with long-term dialysis.

Measurement of complement activation products during dialysis provides a useful indication of the biocompatibility of the membrane. The most sensitive indicator of ongoing activation appears to be measurement of plasma terminal complement complex (TCC) concentration, although measurement of C3adesArg and the C3b,BbP complex may also be of value. The plasma concentration of C5adesArg does not rise significantly because this molecule binds rapidly to cells. The development of membranes that do not activate complement, either by using new materials or by modifiying existing ones, will minimize the problems outlined above and reduce the risk of iatrogenic injury in dialysis patients.

### 10.2.2 Complement and cardiopulmonary bypass

During cardiopulmonary bypass (CPB) blood is passed through an oxygenator. Several strategies are employed for oxygenation but in all devices the blood is exposed to foreign surfaces. Many of the problems encountered are the same as those noted above for haemodialysis. Most oxygenators utilize nylon mesh liners, and this material has been shown to activate complement efficiently *in vitro*. Complement activation occurs on the bioincompatible surface, and increased plasma levels of anaphylatoxins and TCC have been demonstrated during bypass. Circulating erythrocytes and leucocytes become coated with MACs, although the pathological significance of this observation is as yet uncertain.

Leucopenia is not a prominent feature during CPB, probably because the lung, the major site of neutrophil sequestration during haemodialysis, is by definition not perfused. However, at the end of CPB, circulation to the lungs is restored and direct toxic effects of complement fragments and deposition of activated neutrophils occur, which can precipitate pulmonary inflammation and the adult respiratory distress syndrome (see below). Lung inflammation is only one of a spectrum of complications which may follow CPB. Other sequelae include defects in coagulation and inflammatory changes in the kidneys and central nervous system (postperfusion syndrome). Complement activation and neutrophil aggregation may also be, at least in part, responsible for these effects.

A further peak of complement activation appears to accompany postoperative reversal of anticoagulation by infusion of protamine sulphate. The mechanisms of this second phase of activation are uncertain, although classical-pathway activation by protamine–heparin complexes has been reported. Whatever the mechanism, this second wave of activation may contribute to post-CPB tissue injury.

The incidence of life-threatening lung dysfunction following CPB seems to be much higher in children, up to one-third of patients developing severe postoperative pulmonary complications. Oxygenators made of materials which do not significantly activate complement should greatly reduce postoperative morbidity, particularly in this highly susceptible group. As is the case with haemodialysis membranes, complement activation is much reduced upon second or subsequent use of an oxygenator, implying that activating groups on the foreign surface are blocked on first exposure. Prior incubation of oxygenator membranes with plasma proteins may therefore be an economical means of minimizing toxicity. Modification of the methods used to produce and reverse anticoagulation, by preventing the second phase of activation, may provide a simple way of reducing the incidence of complications.

## 10.2.3 Complement and urinary catheters

Although the position is not as technologically advanced as the preceding situations, the issue of biocompatibility is also of relevance to indwelling catheters. Urinary catheters in particular are often left in the urethra for long periods and are in intimate contact with a mucosa which may be inflamed or disrupted. Urethral strictures may occur, particularly when catheters made of latex are used, and it has been suggested that these strictures are caused by catheter toxicity rather than trauma. It has recently been shown that latex catheters, unlike those made of silicon, induce an inflammatory response and neutrophil infiltration *in vivo*, and activate complement directly *in vitro*. Complement activation by bioincompatible catheters may therefore be involved in the formation of urethral strictures as a consequence of postinflammatory scarring.

## 10.3 COMPLEMENT AND THE ADULT RESPIRATORY DISTRESS SYNDROME

The adult respiratory distress syndrome (ARDS) is an acute inflammatory lung disorder of uncertain aetiology which usually follows a major systemic disturbance. ARDS is characterized pathologically by interstitial oedema and cellular infiltration of the lung, and functionally by markedly impaired gas exchange. It is a relatively common complication in critically ill patients, particularly those with severe pulmonary injury or with disseminated bacterial infections, and has a very high incidence of mortality (approaching 95% in some series). The conditions upon which ARDS may supervene are listed in Table 10.2. These illnesses can be broadly divided into two groups: those in which the lung has been damaged directly and severely (gastric aspiration, pneumonia, drowning), and those where the initial insult does not affect the lung (indirect ARDS). In most of this latter group shock occurs, and the development of ARDS is intimately associated with shock. Complement activation plays an important role in most cases of ARDS not caused by direct lung injury.

The primary condition causes widespread complement activation and formation of active complement fragments. The most important fragment in the pathogenesis of ARDS appears to be C5a or its desArg metabolite. Leucopenia, with a particular dirth of neutrophils, is an early feature and is due to C5a/C5adesArg binding to

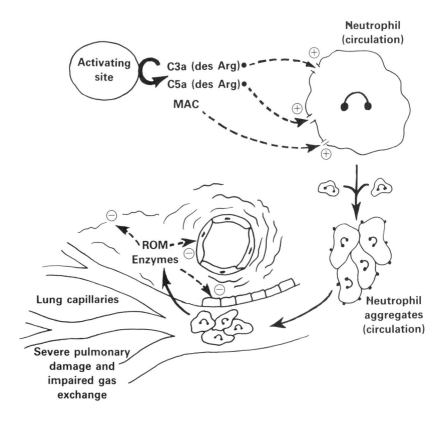

*Figure 10.1* Role of complement and neutrophils in the ARDS.
Complement activation, whatever the primary cause, generates active products which bind to and activate neutrophils. The most important of these active fragments is C5a or its desArg metabolite. Activated neutrophils aggregate and eventually become deposited in the microvasculature of the lung, causing peripheral neutropenia. Continued release of toxic molecules from activated neutrophils damages blood vessels, bronchial elements and supporting tissue in the lung, resulting in pulmonary dysfunction.

and activating neutrophils, thereby increasing cell adherence and aggregation. Aggregates of activated neutrophils become trapped in the capillary network of the lung, thus accounting for the localization of symptoms to this organ. In the lung the activated neutrophils release reactive oxygen metabolites and enzymes which cause tissue destruction (Fig. 10.1). Platelet activation is also a feature of ARDS and may be caused, at least in part, by active products of complement.

Table 10.2 Conditions predisposing to ARDS.

| Condition | Incidence of ARDS (%) |
|---|---|
| Bacterial sepsis | 4* |
| Major trauma | 5 |
| Cardiopulmonary bypass | 2 |
| Burns | 5* |
| Disseminated intravascular coagulation | 22 |
| Severe pneumonia | 12 |
| Gastric aspiration | 36 |

Data in part from Fowler et al., Ann. Intern. Med. **98**, 593–597 (1983).
* Higher incidences have been reported in other studies, probably the result of different definitions of the presenting conditions or of ARDS itself.

Measurement of complement activation may be of particular benefit in the management of severely ill patients at risk of ARDS. Elevated plasma concentrations of C5a, C5adesArg, C3adesArg, C1/C1inh complex, C3b,BbP complex and TCC have all been found consistently in patients with ARDS (Table 10.3). Measurement of TCC levels provides the best discrimination between ARDS patients and severely ill patients without ARDS whatever the underlying pathology. The presence of high concentrations of both the classical-pathway-specific complex (C1/C1inh) and the alternative-pathway-specific complex (C3b,BbP) implies that both activation pathways are involved.

Importantly, it has recently been observed that the increase in plasma concentrations of the activation complexes and the TCC are detectable up to 2 days prior to the onset of clinical symptoms of ARDS. These data further implicate complement in the pathogenesis of the disease and demonstrate that measurement of these complexes is of predictive value in the management of severely ill patients. Identification of impending ARDS may enable appropriate therapy to be instituted early, thereby improving prognosis. A surprising finding in these studies was that an increase in complement activation also occurred prior to resolution of ARDS. It has been suggested that this pre-recovery activation occurs with enhanced removal of pathogens.

This simple concept of complement and neutrophils interacting to cause ARDS has been challenged by several investigators. In particular, the observation that a small number of severely ill

Table 10.3 Usefulness of complement measurement in ARDS due to sepsis.

| Ranking | Parameter | Change[a] | | Discrimination[b] |
|---|---|---|---|---|
| | | With ARDS | Without ARDS | |
| 1 | TCC | 50 | 25 | 0.90* |
| 2 | C1/C1inh | 26 | 20 | 0.68* |
| 3 | C3bBbP | 8 | 6 | 0.53 |
| 4 | C5adesArg | 4 | 2.6 | 0.5 |
| 5 | C3adesArg | 12 | 11 | 0.5 |
| 6 | $CH_{50}$ | 2 | 2 | 0.5 |

Data from Langlois et al., Heart Lung 18, 71–84 (1989).
[a] Fold change, $n$-fold increase over upper limit of normal of parameter.
[b] Discrimination, standard coefficient of discrimination between septicaemic patients with or without ARDS.
* Significant discrimination ($p < 0.01$).

individuals with profound neutropenia have subsequently developed ARDS is hard to reconcile. Nevertheless, the weight of evidence still supports the hypothesis that, in the majority of cases, activation of neutrophils (and perhaps resident lung macrophages) by complement-derived peptides is a major pathogenic factor.

## 10.4 COMPLEMENT AND TRAUMATIC INJURY

Tissue injury and necrosis, however caused, will provide a focus for complement activation. Thus, severe damage to tissues as a result of accidental trauma or of surgical procedures will be accompanied by complement activation. The most serious consequence of this is the potential for ARDS to supervene. Some of the other systemic effects of widespread trauma, including renal failure, may also be due partly to complement activation.

Measurement of complement activation can provide an objective index of the severity of tissue damage which may be particularly useful in the management of unconscious patients or those in whom occult injury is suspected. TCC levels are the most informative single measurement, although determination of the C3a:C3 ratio has recently been shown to be useful. Monitoring complement activation in severely traumatized patients will identify those likely to develop ARDS, enabling early therapeutic intervention.

## 10.5 COMPLEMENT AND ADVERSE DRUG REACTIONS

With the increasing range and potency of therapeutic drugs available, adverse reactions have become increasingly common. These reactions are often characterized by symptoms compatible with an allergic reaction but without evidence of immune dysfunction (pseudoallergic reactions). Many of the symptoms which occur in these reactions could be accounted for by activation of complement and release of active fragments. This possibility has stimulated research on drug-induced complement activation and it has been shown that many therapeutic drugs can activate.

Radiographic contrast media cause pseudoallergic reactions in up to 10% of patients. These compounds activate complement *in vivo* as evidenced by decreased serum complement activity and generation of anaphylactic peptides. The mechanism of activation is complex. Ionic contrast media have been shown to activate C3 directly *in vitro*, whereas nonionic media interfere with control by Factors I and H. However complement activation is initiated, its products may contribute to the observed symptoms.

A variety of other drugs have been shown to influence the complement system. Several anaesthetic agents, including thiopental and phenobarbitone, and antibiotics, such as penicillin, sulphonamides and tetracycline, can all affect complement activity *in vitro*. Dextran, used clinically as a plasma expander, activates complement via the alternative pathway, an effect which may be responsible for the occasional reactions seen on using this drug. The true anticomplementary drugs with a potential therapeutic role in modulating complement activation are discussed in Chapter 12.

## 10.6 FURTHER READING

*Biocompatibility*

Craddock, P. R., Fehr, J., Dalmasso, A. P., Brigham, K. L. and Jacob, H. S. (1977). Hemodialysis leucopenia: pulmonary vascular leucostasis resulting from complement activation by dialyzer cellophane membranes. *J. Clin. Invest.* **59**, 879–888.

Hakim, R. M., Fearon, D. T. and Lazarus, J. M. (1984). Biocompatibility of dialysis membranes: effects of chronic complement activation. *Kidney Int.* **26**, 194–199.

Basile, C. and Drueke, T. (1989). Dialysis membrane biocompatibility. *Nephron* **52**, 113–118.

Chenoweth, D. E., Cooper, S. W., Hugli, T. E., Stewart, R. W., Blackstone,

E. H. and Kirklin, J. W. (1981). Complement activation during cardiopulmonary bypass: evidence for generation of C3a and C5a anaphylatoxins. *N. Engl. J. Med.* **304**, 497–502.

Kirklin, J. K., Westaby, S., Blackstone, E. H., Kirklin, J. W., Chenoweth, D. E. and Pacifico, A. D. (1983). Complement and the damaging effects of cardiopulmonary bypass. *J. Thorac. Cardiovasc. Surg.* **86**, 845–857.

Garred, P., Olsen, J., Mollnes, T. E., Bilde, T. and Glahn, B. E. (1989). Biocompatibility of urinary catheters. Effect on complement activation. *Brit. J. Urol.* **63**, 367–371.

## ARDS

Dal Nogare, A. R. (1989). Adult respiratory distress syndrome. *Am. J. Med. Sci.* **298**, 413-430.

Hammerschmidt, D. E. (1983). Activation of the complement system and of granulocytes in lung injury: the adult respiratory distress syndrome. In: Weissmann, G. (ed.), *Advances in Inflammation Research*. Raven Press, New York, pp. 147–172.

Robins, R., Russ, W., Rasmussen, J. and Clayton, M. (1987). Activation of the complement system in the adult respiratory distress syndrome. *Am. Rev. Resp. Dis.* **135**, 651–658.

Langlois, P. F. and Gawryl, M. S. (1988). Complement activation occurs through both classical and alternative pathways prior to onset and resolution of adult respiratory distress syndrome. *Clin. Immunol. Immunopathol.* **47**, 152–163.

## Drug reactions

Rother, U. (1988). Adverse reactions to drugs. In: Rother, K. and Till, G. O. (eds), *The Complement System*. Springer, Berlin, pp. 511–519.

# CHAPTER ELEVEN
# Complement in Other Diseases

## 11.1 INTRODUCTION

In the preceding chapters the role of complement in several groups of diseases has been described. Inevitably, many interesting conditions were not covered because they did not fit into any of the groups chosen. This chapter is therefore a *pot-pourri* of pathologies in which complement has been implicated. As emphasized in the preceding chapters, in most of the conditions described here complement is just one factor contributing to a complex, multifactorial pathogenesis.

## 11.2 COMPLEMENT IN CARDIOVASCULAR DISEASE

### 11.2.1 Atheroma and complement

Evidence for an involvement of complement in the pathogenesis of atheroma has been provided by the identification of complement components and activation products in the walls of diseased vessels. C3, C4, C3c, C3d, S-protein and the membrane attack complex (MAC) have all been detected in damaged areas of the vessel wall, and a quantitative study has shown that the degree of MAC deposition correlates with the severity of arterial damage (Fig. 11.1). MAC is present in areas of intimal thickening and in fibrous

## Complement in Other Diseases

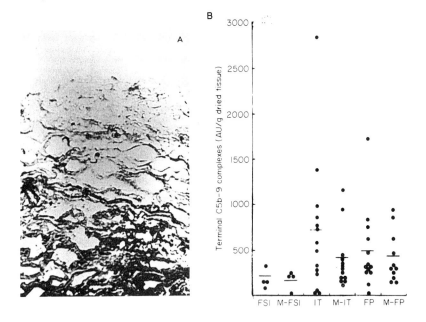

*Figure 11.1* Membrane attack complex deposition in atheroma.
(A) Atheromatous arterial wall stained for MAC (black staining) using an antineo-antigenic antibody. Control normal artery contained only small amounts of MAC. Magnification × 250. Reproduced from Niculescu et al., *Clin. Exp. Immunol.* **69**, 477–482 (1987). (B) MACs eluted from different regions of atheromatous vessel wall and then quantified in a specific ELISA assay. High concentrations of MAC were eluted from fibrous plaques (FP) and from intimal thickenings (IT), and lower amounts from intimal fatty streaks (FS-I). From Rus et al., *Clin. Exp. Immunol.* **65**, 66–72 (1986).

plaques, and it has been suggested that the complement system is activated at these sites by deposits of crystalline cholesterol. Activation of complement may then damage resident cells of the arterial wall or infiltrating macrophages, exacerbating the disease process.

Further evidence of an involvement of complement is provided by several animal studies. Complement depletion of rats using cobra venom factor (CVF) renders them resistant to vitamin-D2-induced atheroma, and the severity of cholesterol-induced atheroma is markedly reduced in rabbits depleted of complement or deficient in C6.

It should be emphasized that complement deposition can also be detected in the walls of apparently normal large blood vessels from virtually all individuals over the age of 30, although the extent of deposition is much less than in atheromatous vessels. It has been suggested that these deposits are indicative of early atheromatous changes not detectable by other means.

## 11.2.2 Myocardial infarction and complement

Although the primary pathology in myocardial infarction (MI) — ischaemia of cardiac muscle — is certain, a role of complement in the enlargement or extension of infarcts immediately following the acute event has been suggested. Complement deposition within and at the periphery of infarcted areas has been demonstrated. The MAC is present on necrotic cells and on prenecrotic cells at the edge of the lesion, and it has been postulated that MAC-induced calcium influx is at least in part responsible for muscle cell damage. The mechanism of complement activation on cardiac cells is uncertain but damaged cardiac cells activate complement directly *in vitro* via both the classical and alternative pathways. The activating factor released from the damaged cells appears to be a mitochondrial component which binds C1 and initiates classical-pathway activation in the absence of antibody. Activation of complement by dead or dying cells might therefore initiate a vicious cycle of increased tissue destruction by damaging surrounding cells directly and also by the recruitment of phagocytic cells, which release enzymes and other toxic molecules.

Evidence from animal models again supports the contention that complement contributes to tissue damage in MI. Deposits of complement are found in experimentally induced infarcts in a variety of animals, and complement depletion using CVF in rats and in baboons reduces the size of the experimentally induced lesions and inhibits phagocyte infiltration.

Although substantial evidence exists for local activation of complement in acute MI, measurement of systemic complement does not reveal significant activation, implying that activation is restricted to the infarct. Measurement of serum activation products is therefore unlikely to be of any help in the management of patients with MI.

## 11.3. AUTOIMMUNE ENDOCRINE DISEASE AND COMPLEMENT

In several endocrine diseases autoantibodies directed against cells or products of a specific organ are central to pathogenesis. Autoantibodies stimulate or damage the target organ either directly or by recruiting immune effector systems. The involvement of cell-mediated immunity has been well studied in many of these diseases, but the possible role of complement has attracted scant attention. A cursory glance at the preceding chapters provides ample evidence that complement may contribute to pathogenesis in autoimmune diseases, yet so far its relevance to endocrine diseases has been closely examined in only one group of conditions.

### 11.3.1 Autoimmune thyroid disease and complement

A variety of immunological abnormalities have been described in the two principal forms of autoimmune thyroid disease, Graves' disease and Hashimoto's thyroiditis. Autoantibodies against thyroglobulin, thyroid microsomal antigen (M) and the thyroid-stimulating hormone (TSH) receptor have been found and a subset of anti-TSH receptor antibodies directly stimulate the thyroid cells to induce the hyperthyroidism of Graves' disease. The role of the other antibodies is less certain. Antibodies against the M antigen have been shown to be complement-fixing *in vitro* and these antibodies have been implicated in thyroid tissue destruction.

Direct evidence of complement activation in these diseases has been provided by localization of C1, C3, C9 and recently the MAC in thyroid tissue. All the components and the MAC were deposited in association with the follicular basement membrane in both diseases. MAC deposition on the basement membrane was more evident in Graves' disease, but in Hashimoto's thyroid MAC was also present in the lymphocytic foci (Fig. 11.2). The levels of terminal complement (TCC) in the plasma of patients were elevated to a similar extent in the two diseases. The C1/C1 inhibitor complex — an indicator of classical-pathway activation — was also present in increased amounts in both diseases, although the levels in Graves' disease were higher (Fig. 11.2).

The contribution to pathology made by complement activation in thyroid disease is still not clear. Complement may be responsible for cellular infiltration (via the active fragments C3a and C5a) and for thyroid cell death (via the MAC) in Hashimoto's thyroiditis. In

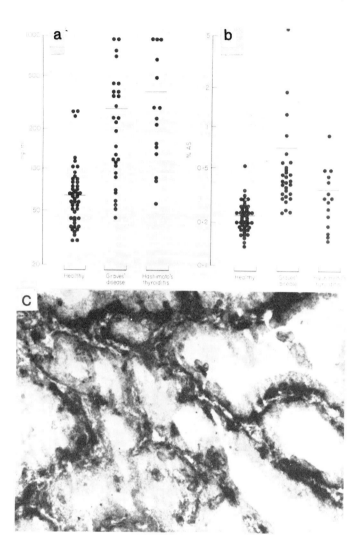

Figure 11.2 Complement activation in autoimmune thyroid disease.
(a) Serum terminal complement complex (TCC) and (b) C1/C1 inhibitor (C1/C1inh) levels in patients with untreated Graves' disease and with Hashimoto's thyroiditis. Each horizontal bar represents the mean. The levels of TCCs were significantly elevated ($p < 0.001$) in both patient groups but C1/C1inh levels were significantly elevated ($p < 0.001$) only in patients with Graves' disease. (c) Staining of Graves' thyroid tissue with MAC-specific antibody. MAC deposition is present on the basement membrane of the thyroid follicles. Control tissues showed no staining. Magnification × 480). Reproduced from Weetman et al., Clin. Exp. Immunol. 77, 25–30 (1989), with permission.

Graves' disease, however, infiltration and cell death are not prominent features. Here the MAC may act nonlethally on the thyroid cells to stimulate the release of inflammatory molecules, thus potentiating inflammation and tissue injury.

### 11.3.2 Other endocrine diseases and complement

As noted above, the role of complement in other autoimmune endocrine diseases has yet to be examined systematically. In all these diseases specific autoantibodies are present, often recognizing cell surface determinants. If these antibodies can activate complement then the potential for complement-induced tissue damage exists. However, little is known about the complement fixing activities of endocrine autoantibodies.

Complement fixing islet-cell antibodies have been described in Type I diabetes mellitus and the appearance of these antibodies has been shown to be closely related to the onset of clinical disease. Thereafter, complement fixing antibodies disappear from the serum, implying that they are involved in beta cell destruction during the genesis of the disease. Recently, elevated levels of the C1/C1 inhibitor complex have been demonstrated in newly diagnosed Type I diabetics, further implicating antibody-mediated classical-pathway activation in islet cell destruction. Examination of complement activation in diabetics is thus complicated because it is likely to occur only at disease onset and may perhaps be undetectable by the time the disease becomes clinically apparent.

### 11.4. COMPLEMENT AND INFLAMMATORY BOWEL DISEASE

The inflammatory bowel diseases (IBD), Crohn's disease and ulcerative colitis, are relatively common debilitating diseases of unknown aetiology which differ principally in that they affect different areas of the bowel. A wide variety of pathogenic factors have been implicated in IBD and the current consensus of opinion favours autoimmunity as the underlying cause. Immunoglobulin is produced within the diseased mucosa and locally synthesized IgG is directed in part against intestinal microorganisms and mucosal epithelium. Immune complexes form within the mucosa, particularly at the epithelial basement membrane, and provide a focus for complement activation. Evidence for ongoing complement activation in IBD has been provided by localization of complement components and activation products in the bowel wall. C3 breakdown products and the MAC are present in the walls of submucosal vessels and in the muscular layers of the gut wall in Crohn's disease and in ulcerative colitis, and a role for the chemotactic peptides and the MAC in propagating inflammation has been suggested.

Further evidence that immune complex formation and complement activation are important in the pathogenesis of IBD has been derived from animal studies. In rabbits, deposition of preformed immune complexes in the colon induces a severe colitis which clinically and histologically resembles human IBD. The effects of decomplementation on the course of this experimental disease have not been investigated.

Coeliac disease is a malabsorption syndrome characterized histologically by villous atrophy and low-grade inflammation in the wall of the small intestine, particularly the jejunum. The primary cause of this disease is known, gluten in the diet exerting a toxic effect on the intestinal mucosa. What is less certain is the mechanism by which toxicity is mediated. Substantial evidence indicates that individuals with coeliac disease mount an immune response to gluten. Immunoglobulin, particularly IgA, is synthesized in the gut wall and, in patients with active disease, complement is deposited in the lamina propria or on the basement membrane. Following treatment of coeliac disease by removing gluten from the diet complement deposits are no longer detectable. The association of coeliac disease with dermatitis herpetiformis and the involvement of complement in this disease are discussed in Section 9.2.3.

## 11.5 COMPLEMENT IN HAEMOLYTIC ANAEMIA AND THROMBOCYTOPENIA

Haemolytic anaemia may be caused by any event which shortens the survival time of erythrocytes. In the broadest terms this may result from abnormalities in the erythrocyte itself or from extrinsic factors. In the first category, complement plays a significant role only in those diseases where the primary defect results in an increased susceptibility to lysis, exemplified by paroxysmal nocturnal haemoglobinuria (Section 4.3.5.4). In the second category, the commonest primary factors are abnormal immune responses or toxins (drugs, poisons, etc.) and complement is in many instances involved in erythrocyte removal. This section first describes the physiological processes of erythrocyte clearance in order to clarify the abnormalities occurring in disease.

Thrombocytopenia is caused either by a diminished production of platelets or by a decrease in platelet survival. The commonest causes of decreased platelet survival are exposure to drugs and the presence of antiplatelet autoantibodies (autoimmune thrombocytopenia). Occasionally, autoimmune thrombocytopenia and haemolytic anaemia occur together (Evans' syndrome).

### 11.5.1 Complement and erythrocyte clearance

The average lifespan of an erythrocyte in the circulation is 120 days and in the normal situation the vast majority of cells are cleared within a few days of this mean. Complement is involved in the removal of senescent erythrocytes. During ageing, sialic acid is shed from the membrane, rendering the cell surface more amenable to alternative pathway activation. Recent evidence suggests that decay accelerating factor and perhaps other specific complement inhibitory proteins are also lost from the erythrocyte surface during ageing, further enhancing the potential for complement activation. Deposition of C3 fragments on senescent erythrocytes facilitates interaction with complement-receptor-rich cells in the reticuloendothelial system (RES) and subsequent clearance.

### 11.5.2 Complement and autoimmune haemolytic anaemia

Autoantibodies against antigens present on the erythrocyte surface can cause haemolysis. In the majority of cases the antibodies are IgG and react optimally at 37°C (warm-reacting antibodies). Coating of erythrocytes with IgG antibody will itself render the cells susceptible to clearance by binding to Fc receptors on cells in the RES. However, the majority of these antibodies are complement fixing, and binding of fragments of C3 and C4 greatly enhances removal. The presence of complement fixing antierythrocyte antibodies can be confirmed using antisera against C3 or C4 which cause agglutination of erythrocytes bearing fragments of these components (Coombs' test). Complement-mediated lysis is rarely seen in autoimmune haemolytic anaemia caused by IgG antibodies, probably because of the presence on erythrocytes of membrane proteins which protect cells against lysis by homologous complement (see Section 1.3.4.3). A minority of patients with autoimmune haemolytic anaemia mediated by IgG antibody are Coombs' test negative, indicating that complement activation has not occurred. This failure to activate complement is probably related to the sparsity of the antigen against which the particular antibody is directed. Even in these Coombs' negative anaemias, more sensitive techniques often detect small amounts of C3 fragments on the erythrocyte surface — complement may therefore still contribute to clearance.

A second group of autoimmune haemolytic anaemias is caused by antibodies which bind optimally to the erythrocyte at low temperatures (cold-reacting antibodies). These antibodies bind to erythrocytes in the peripheral circulation, where if the external environment is cold the blood temperature may fall to around 30°C, and dissociate on rewarming to 37°C. Cold-reacting antibodies are almost invariably IgM antibodies, usually of anti-I specificity. These antibodies activate complement via the classical pathway very efficiently, and therefore cause lysis of a significant proportion of attacked erythrocytes. Unlysed cells are coated with fragments of C3 and C4 but the cold-reacting antibodies dissociate from erythrocytes in the warmer central circulation. In the RES these complement-coated erythrocytes bind to fixed macrophages, but in the absence of surface immunoglobulin clearance is much less efficient. Processing of complement fragments occurs and a large proportion of the bound erythrocytes are released intact but coated with the opsonically inactive C3d fragment (Section 2.3; Fig. 11.3). In paroxysmal cold haemoglobinuria, a cold-reacting IgG antibody with anti-P specificity (Donath–Landsteiner antibody) is present which, unlike most IgG antierythrocyte antibodies, is extremely efficient at inducing complement dependent haemolysis.

Both warm-reacting and cold-reacting antibody-mediated haemolytic anaemias may occur in isolation (idiopathic) or may be associated with other autoimmune diseases, with viral infections or with lymphoid malignancy. In this last case a monoclonal autoantibody may be present.

### 11.5.3 Complement and transfusion reactions

Transfusion reactions occur as a result of the binding of isoimmune antibodies to the transfused erythrocytes. The mechanisms of erythrocyte removal are identical to those described above for autoimmune haemolytic anaemias. Antibodies which fix complement efficiently — those directed against the major blood group

## 188 Complement in Other Diseases

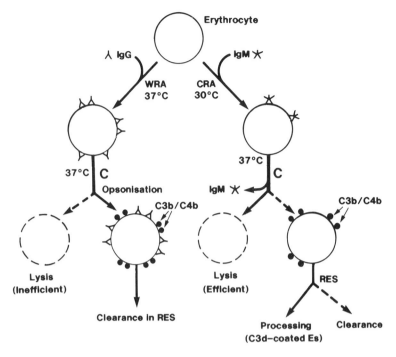

*Figure 11.3* Complement and autoimmune haemolytic anaemia.
Warm-reacting antierythrocyte antibodies (WRA, IgG) bind at 37°C and fix complement. Most cells are then efficiently cleared in the reticuloendothelial system (RES), direct lysis accounting for only a small proportion of erythrocyte loss. Cold-reacting antibodies (CRA, IgM) bind at low temperatures in the periphery and dissociate on warming to 37°C. Prior to dissociating they efficiently fix complement, a large proportion of attacked cells being lysed. In the absence of surface antibody, clearance in the RES is inefficient, but processing of cell-bound C3 fragments occurs with the release of C3d-coated erythrocytes into the circulation.

antigens — cause immediate haemolysis of the transfused cells. Those directed against minor blood group antigens fix complement sublytically, enhancing erythrocyte clearance in the RES.

### 11.5.4 Complement in drug-induced haemolysis

Drug-induced anaemias are usually a consequence of direct toxic damage to erythrocytes or precursor cells. However, haemolytic anaemia may also occur as a result of an immune response to a drug. A variety of agents, including the anti-arrhythmic drug quinidine, have been shown to cause haemolysis in this way. Soluble drug-containing immune complexes form and bind to erythrocytes, providing a focus for complement activation on the erythrocyte surface. Depending on the degree of activation, lysis may ensue rapidly or the affected erythrocyte may be removed in the RES.

### 11.5.5 Complement and platelets

Platelets, like erythrocytes, have a finite lifespan in the circulation. The average lifespan of a platelet is about 9 days, after which it is removed in the spleen or liver. During ageing the cells lose surface sialic acid, and complement activation probably plays a part in the removal of senescent platelets. Specific complement inhibiting proteins are present on the membranes but their role in determining platelet survival has not been investigated.

Complement has also been implicated in platelet activation. Nonlethal complement attack causes aggregation of platelets and release of histamine and enzymes *in vitro*. Assembly of the complete MAC is required for activation. An involvement of the MAC in platelet activation *in vivo* is suggested by the finding that some individuals with deficiencies of terminal complement components have abnormal platelet function. Calcium influx via the MAC has been suggested to be the trigger to activation *in vivo*. The anaphylactic fragment C3a has also been implicated in platelet activation but its importance *in vivo* is uncertain.

### 11.5.6 Complement in autoimmune thrombocytopenia

Idiopathic thrombocytopenic purpura (ITP) is an autoimmune disease in which antiplatelet autoantibodies bind to and initiate destruction of platelets. The autoantibodies are usually IgG and are, in the majority of cases, complement-fixing. Platelets from patients with ITP have detectable amounts of IgG and/or C3 fragments on their surfaces although the exact nature of the bound fragments is not known. The relative contributions of enhanced clearance in the RES (a consequence of bound IgG/C3) and of direct lysis by the MAC to the development of thrombocytopenia have not been assessed. Platelet activation by nonlethal amounts of the MAC may, by stimulating aggregation, also contribute to the development of thrombocytopenia.

## 190 Complement in Other Diseases

### 11.6 COMPLEMENT IN PULMONARY DISEASE

The anatomy and pathology of the lung alveolus and the kidney glomerulus are similar in several respects. In both an exposed epithelial cell layer is separated from the vascular compartment by a functionally and structurally important basement membrane and endothelial cell layers, and immune complex deposition on or close to the basement membrane is a common pathological finding. However, in comparison with renal disease (Chapter 6), the role of complement in pulmonary disease has been much less studied. Nevertheless, complement mediated lung injury has been implicated in several types of pulmonary disease, including hypersensitivity reactions and pulmonary fibrosis. Several animal models of human lung diseases have been useful in this context. Acute pulmonary alveolitis is induced in rats by the formation of immune complexes *in situ* in the lung. An acute inflammatory reaction develops in and around the alveolus which resembles that seen in human interstitial pneumonitis. Depletion of either C3 (using CVF) or neutrophils ameliorates the experimental disease, suggesting that complement activation, by releasing chemotactic fragments, attracts neutrophils into the pulmonary interstitium where they damage surrounding tissue (see Fig. 10.1). A direct role of complement in pulmonary damage has also been suggested. The MAC has been shown to cause disruption of the pulmonary basement membrane *in vitro* and damage to this important structure has been implicated in many diseases.

The role of complement activation in the adult respiratory distress syndrome is described in Section 10.3. The pulmonary diseases in which complement activation is implicated, and the supporting evidence, are summarized in Table 11.1.

### 11.7 COMPLEMENT IN PRE-ECLAMPSIA

Pre-eclampsia is a common complication of pregnancy and is characterized by hypertension, oedema, proteinuria and placental insufficiency. The condition is commoner in first pregnancies and rarely presents prior to the 30th week of pregnancy. The aetiology of pre-eclampsia has attracted much investigation but remains uncertain. An immunological basis has been suggested by several pieces of evidence. High concentrations of circulating immune complexes are present in the circulation which decline rapidly after parturition. Immune complexes are also present in the placenta and

*Table 11.1* Complement and pulmonary disease.

| Disease | Evidence |
|---|---|
| Chronic bronchitis | C3 deposits in alveolar septa |
| Bronchial asthma | C3 deposits on alveolar basement membrane |
| Sarcoidosis | C3 deposits in and around granulomas |
| 'Heroin lung' | C3 deposits in alveolar septa |
| Goodpasture's syndrome | C3 deposits on alveolar basement membrane |
| Adult respiratory distress syndrome | Marked systemic complement activation, C5a implicated in pathogenesis |
| Experimental lung injury in rats | Complement dependence of lung injury (CVF treatment protects) |

recently it has been shown that complement activation products, including the MAC, are present in greater amounts in pre-eclamptic placentae than in normal placentae of the same gestational age. Whether complement is involved directly in the causation of either renal dysfunction or of placental failure in pre-eclampsia remains to be determined.

## 11.8 FURTHER READING

*Cardiovascular disease*

Jacob, H. S. (1983). Complement-mediated leucoembolization: a mechanism of tissue damage during extracorporeal perfusions, myocardial infarction and in shock — a review. *Qt. J. Med.* **207**, 289–296.

McManus, L. M., Kolb, W. P., Crawford, M. H., O'Rourke, R. A., Grover, F. L. and Pinckard, R. N. (1983). Complement localization in ischaemic baboon myocardium. *Lab. Invest.* **48**, 436–447.

Schafer, H., Mathey, D., Hugo, F. and Bhakdi, S. (1986). Deposition of the terminal C5b–9 complex in infarcted areas of human myocardium. *J. Immunol.* **137**, 1945–1949.

Niculescu, F., Rus, H. G. and Vlaicu, R. (1987). Immunohistochemical localization of C5b–9, S-protein, C3d and apolipoprotein B in human arterial tissues with atherosclerosis. *Atherosclerosis* **65**, 1–11.

*Haemolytic anaemia and thrombocytopenia*

Nydegger, U. E. and Kazatchkine, M. D. (1983). The role of complement in immune clearance of blood cells. *Springer Semin. Immunopathol.* **6**, 373–398.

Leddy, J. P. and Rosenfeld, S. I. (1986). Role of complement in hemolytic anemia and thrombocytopenia. In: Ross, G. D. (ed.), *Immunobiology of the Complement System*. Academic Press, London, pp. 213–236.

*Others*

Weetman, A. P., Cohen, S. B., Oleesky, D. A. and Morgan, B. P. (1989). Terminal complement complexes and C1/C1 inhibitor complexes in autoimmune thyroid disease. *Clin. Exp. Immunol.* **77**, 25–30.

Halstensen, T. S., Mollnes, T. E., Fausa, O. and Brandtzaeg, P. (1989). Deposits of terminal complement complex (TCC) in muscularis mucosae and submucosal vessels in ulcerative colitis and Crohn's disease of the colon. *Gut* **30**, 361–366.

Johnson, K. J. and Ward, P. A. (1974). Acute immunologic pulmonary alveolitis. *J. Clin. Invest.* **54**, 349–357.

Kopp, W. C. and Burrel, R. (1982). Evidence for antibody-independent binding of the terminal complement component to alveolar basement membrane. *Clin. Immunol. Immunopathol.* **23**, 10–21.

CHAPTER TWELVE

# Complement Measurement and Potential for Therapeutic Manipulation

## 12.1 INTRODUCTION

The preceding chapters have described the important features and biological activities of the complement system, its protective roles in neutralizing pathogenic organisms and in maintaining immune complexes in solution, and the evidence implicating complement as a causative factor in a wide range of diseases. A wealth of experimental and clinical data has been reviewed and the reader should now be persuaded, if persuasion were needed, of the importance of this effector system. The sheer number of conditions in which complement plays a part makes it unlikely that measurements of complement activation will be of much help in diagnosis. However, assessment of activation may be extremely useful as an objective measure of disease activity and as an indicator of response to treatment. Methods for measurement of complement activation and therapeutic manipulation of the complement system are therefore of potential relevance to all clinicians, not just to the select few. The first aim of this chapter is to provide a concise and up-to-date account of the currently available assays for complement activity and activation, together with their relative merits and demerits. The second aim is to outline the strategies which have been employed or suggested specifically in order to modulate complement activation *in vivo*. It is hoped that an increased awareness of the potential role of complement in many diseases, together with the availability of better assays and therapeutic agents, will contribute to a reduction in morbidity.

## 12.2 ASSAYS OF COMPLEMENT ACTIVITY AND ACTIVATION

Complement assays are broadly divisible into functional assays which measure the activity of the whole system or of selected components, and immunochemical assays which measure the amount of a particular component by using specific antibodies. Both types of assays are discussed in the following sections. A third type of investigation which is of clinical importance is the determination of allotypic variants. This subject was discussed in Chapter 3 and is not reiterated here.

### 12.2.1 Measurement of functional complement activity

Haemolytic assays have been the cornerstone of complement measurement for over 50 years and even today they provide an extremely useful screening procedure, particularly when investigating possible complement deficiencies. These assays may be used to assess separately the integrity of the classical and alternative activation pathways and the terminal pathway, and can also be modified to measure the functional activity of specific components. Classical-pathway activity in serum is usually assessed by measurement of lysis of antibody-sensitized sheep erythrocytes either in suspension or in agarose gel (haemolysis-in-gel assay). Alternative-pathway activity is measured using unsensitized guinea pig or rabbit erythrocytes in a magnesium-EDTA (calcium-free) buffer. In either case, the amount of test serum required to cause 50% haemolysis of the erythrocytes is compared to pooled normal serum and the relative activity calculated. The results are expressed as a percentage of the lytic activity in normal serum ($CH_{50}$ for the classical pathway, $AH_{50}$ for the alternative). Detection of low or absent lytic activity in either or both of these assays provides important clues to the underlying problem and directs further investigations in the appropriate direction (Table 12.1).

The haemolytic activity of individual components was until recently measured using sera in which specific components had been inactivated by physical or chemical means. These reagents have now largely been superseded by sera congenitally deficient in or immunochemically depleted of the component of interest. For example, C8 activity in a test serum can be assessed by adding portions to serum specifically depleted of C8 and measuring restoration of lytic activity.

Table 12.1 Haemolytic complement activity and component assays.

|  | $CH_{50}$ | $AH_{50}$ | C3 | C4 | FB |
|---|---|---|---|---|---|
| CP deficiency (C1, C4, C2) | ↓↓↓ | N | | | |
| AP deficiency (FB, P, FD) | N | ↓↓↓ | | | |
| TP deficiency (C5–C9) | ↓↓↓ | ↓↓↓ | | | |
| C3 deficiency | ↓↓↓ | ↓↓↓ | | | |
| CP activation | ↓ | N | ↓ | ↓ | N |
| AP activation | N | ↓ | ↓ | N | ↓ |
| Combined activation | ↓ | ↓ | ↓ | ↓ | ↓ |

CP, Classical pathway; AP, alternative pathway; FB, FD, Factors B and D; P, properdin; ↓, reduced; ↓↓↓, markedly reduced or absent.

Recently, a number of technical improvements on the standard haemolytic assays have been described. Microassays are now commonly employed which require only small amounts of sample. Attempts have been made to remove the requirement for animal erythrocytes, which can vary greatly from batch to batch. In particular, several methods have now been reported which measure complement lytic activity by determining the release of a fluorescent dye from liposomes coated with antibody. These liposome lysis assays are highly sensitive and the reagents are very stable, offering potential advantages over traditional haemolytic techniques.

A detailed description of the methodology of lytic assays is beyond the scope of this book. Several excellent accounts of the techniques of complement assay exist and are listed at the end of the chapter.

## 12.2.2 Immunochemical measurement of native components

Measurements of the plasma levels of C3, C4 and Factor B remain the mainstay of clinical complement assay in most centres. The components are measured using specific antisera in a variety of immunoprecipitation methods — radial immunodiffusion, rocket immunoelectrophoresis, immunonephelometry, etc. Measurement of these three components, particularly if accompanied by haemolytic assays of total complement activity, enables complement activation to be detected and the pathway(s) involved to be identified (Table 12.1). The assays are relatively simple to perform but provide only very limited information. Levels of individual components merely reflect the balance between synthesis and catabolism, and are influenced by many factors. They are consequently insensitive to minor degrees of complement activation and to small but clinically important fluctuations.

Immunochemical measurements of other components are also of limited value. Measurement of specific components is necessary to confirm a suspected deficiency, but outside this situation these assays are unlikely to be of much clinical relevance. Measurement of individual components, particularly C9, has occasionally been shown to provide a useful clinical index in a few diseases (Section 7.3.2), but even in these situations the sensitive and specific assays described below are likely to be more clinically useful.

### 12.2.3 The concept of neoantigens

During complement activation protein molecules are cleaved and form multimolecular complexes. Both of these phenomena cause conformational changes in the component proteins, resulting in the exposure of areas of the molecule which are buried within the native protein. These newly exposed areas thus represent specific markers for a given fragment or complex, and antibodies which recognize these 'neoantigenic determinants' will detect only the corresponding fragment or complex. Monoclonal and polyclonal antibodies which recognize neoantigenic determinants on several of the fragments and complexes formed during complement activation have recently been described and have been utilized to develop highly specific assays for complement activation. The principles underlying the exposure of neoantigenic determinants and production of antineoantigenic antibodies are illustrated in Fig. 12.1.

### 12.2.4 Measurement of complement fragments

During complement activation a number of small and large fragments are released to the fluid phase (Chapter 2). Measurement of these fragments in biological fluids provides a highly specific means of identifying and quantifying activation *in vivo*. The utility of

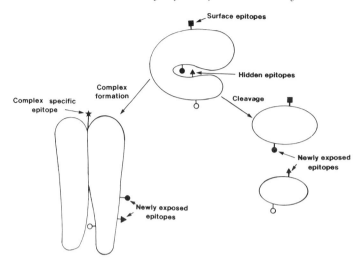

*Figure 12.1* The concept of neoantigens.
A globular serum protein contains surface epitopes accessible to antibodies and internal epitopes which are hidden and not available for antibody binding. These hidden epitopes may become exposed upon unfolding of the molecule during complex formation or following cleavage, and are consequently available for binding of specific antibodies (antineoantigenic antibodies). Neoantigenic epitopes may also be formed on multimolecular complexes at areas of apposition of two proteins, each contributing to the formation of the epitope.

the different fragments as indicators of activation is dependent on several factors: (1) the ease of production of specific antibodies against the fragment; (2) the amount produced; (3) the stability of the fragment in the circulation; and (4) the stability of the fragment in plasma *in vitro*. Stability of the fragments both *in vivo* and *in vitro*, and continued activation of complement in plasma samples, have proven to be the major obstacles to the widespread use of these measurements in assessing complement activation.

The small (about 10 kDa) anaphylactic and chemotactic fragments C3a, C4a and C5a are rapidly converted into their inactive desArg metabolites by anaphylatoxin inactivator (Section 2.2.1). C5adesArg binds avidly to leucocyte receptors and is thus present in plasma at extremely low concentrations (below 10 ng/ml). C3adesArg and C4adesArg are less avidly bound and are therefore present in higher concentrations (above 100 ng/ml). Competitive radioimmunoassays capable of detecting anaphylatoxins in clinical samples have been available for several years. These assays measure the competitive binding of radiolabelled and unlabelled (sample) anaphylatoxin to an antibody, and all require prior processing to remove the parent molecule (C3, C4, C5). Recently, highly specific monoclonal antibodies recognizing neoantigenic determinants expressed only on C3adesArg and not on C3 have been described, enabling rapid, nonisotopic assays to be performed on unprocessed samples. The major limiting factor in all anaphylatoxin assays is that minor degrees of complement activation *in vitro*, remote from the buffering leucocytes, cause marked increases in the measured values. Taking samples into the calcium-chelating anticoagulant EDTA, storage on ice and prompt assay all help to minimize activation but do not completely abolish it. Recently, a new protease inhibitor has been developed which is claimed greatly to reduce *in vitro* activation (nafamostat mesylate, Amersham). If these claims are substantiated, the use of this or similar inhibitors, together with specific antibodies, will simplify and improve anaphylatoxin assays, making them suitable for routine diagnostic use.

Apart from the C3a fragment, the split products of C3 include C3b, C3bi, C3c and C3d,g (Fig. 1.5). Measurement of the plasma levels of any of these fragments could therefore be used to provide an index of complement activation. The fragment C3d can be measured in plasma using antisera against C3d following precipitation of uncleaved C3 either by polyethylene glycol or by immunoprecipitation with anti-C3c antiserum. Precipitation of intact C3 can be achieved in the first phase of a two-phase immunoelectrophoresis procedure, obviating the need for sample processing (double-decker rocket electrophoresis; Fig. 12.2). Recently, monoclonal antibodies have been described which recognize neoantigenic determinants expressed only in cleaved C3, enabling the development of assays which can quantify C3 conversion without the requirement for a separation step.

Fragmentation of C4 follows the same course as that of C3, and the fragments released are structurally similar (Fig. 2.4). Assays for split products of C4 have developed along similar lines to those described above for C3. A monoclonal antibody which recognizes a neoantigenic determinant in the C4d fragment has been produced and used to develop a simple and specific ELISA assay for this fragment.

Factor B is cleaved upon activation, into Ba and Bb fragments. Assays for both fragments have been established using specific antisera. Ba has been measured by double-decker immunoelectrophoresis using antiserum against Bb in the first gel (precipitates Factor B and Bb) and specific antiserum against Ba in the second gel. Recently, monoclonal antibodies specific for the two fragments have been produced and used to develop specific assays.

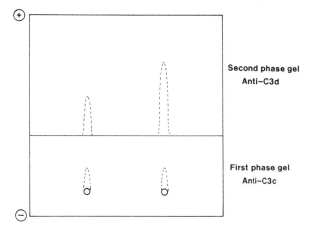

*Figure 12.2* Double-decker rocket immunoelectrophoresis.
A schematic representation of the principles of this useful technique. Serum samples are placed in the wells on the plate and are then electrophoresed through a first gel containing antiserum which recognizes the intact molecule but not the fragment of interest. In this example, anti-C3c antiserum precipitates native C3 and the fragments containing C3c. The C3d fragment is then detected by its precipitation in the second gel which contains antiserum which recognizes C3d. Cross-reactivity of this second antiserum with other parts of the C3 molecule is inconsequential because they are precipitated in the first gel.

All measurements of complement fragments are influenced by complement activation *in vitro*, and care must be taken to minimize this. The relative effects of *in vitro* activation appear to be less for the larger fragments such as C3d than for the anaphylatoxins, where small amounts of activation may greatly alter the measured concentrations. The current assays for complement fragments are summarized in Table 12.2.

### 12.2.5 Measurement of complement activation complexes

Each of the three pathways which constitute the complement system produces a specific fluid-phase activation complex. Two-site assays have been developed for each of the complexes utilizing antibodies against two different constituents of the complex, providing highly sensitive and specific results.

#### 12.2.5.1 Activation complex of the classical pathway
The fluid-phase activation complex of the classical pathway is the

Table 12.2 Measurement of complement fragments.

| Fragment | Assay methods | Comments |
| --- | --- | --- |
| Anaphylatoxins (C3a, C4a, C5a) | Radioimmunoassay, neoantigen-based ELISA | Very low concentrations in plasma, *in vitro* activation gives false elevations |
| Large C3 fragment (C3d,g, C3c, C3b) | Double-decker RIE, precipitation/nephelometry, neoantigen-based ELISA | Higher concentrations, less affected by *in vitro* activation, new assays using antineo very reliable |
| Large C4 fragments (C4b, C4c, C4d) | As above | As above: specific index of CP activation |
| Factor B fragments | Double-decker RIE, immunoprecipitation/ELISA | New assays using specific MoAbs reliable: specific index of AP activation |

CP, Classical pathway; AP, alternative pathway; ELISA, enzyme-linked immunosorbent assay; RIE, rocket immunoelectrophoresis; Antineo, antineoantigenic antibody; MoAb, monoclonal antibody.

C1/C1 inhibitor (C1/C1inh) complex. The complex is formed during inactivation of C1 and contains two molecules of C1 inhibitor together with one molecule each of C1r and C1s, C1q remaining attached to the activating surface. Using antibodies against C1s and C1inh, a specific and sensitive ELISA assay capable of measuring C1/C1inh levels in plasma has been developed. Anti-C1s immobilized on the plate captures the C1/C1inh complex (and any free C1s) from the sample, and the bound complex is subsequently detected by anti-C1inh (Fig. 12.3). Working assays have been produced using commercially available polyclonal antibodies. No monoclonal or antineoantigenic antibody based assays have yet been described.

#### 12.2.5.2 Activation complex of the alternative pathway

The fluid-phase activation complex of the alternative pathway is the C3b,BbP complex. This complex is detected using antibodies directed against properdin (P) and C3. Anti-P antibody immobilized on the plate captures the C3b,BbP complex (and any free P) from the sample, and the bound complex is detected subsequently using anti-C3 (Fig. 12.3). Assays so far described utilize polyclonal antibodies against native components. Considerable potential exists for using complex-specific (antineoantigenic) monoclonal antibodies in these assays.

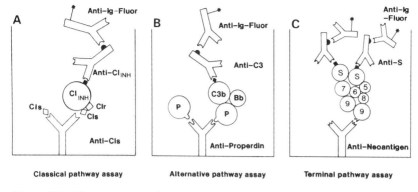

*Figure 12.3* Measurement of complement activation complexes.
A schematic representation of the ELISA assay protocols for: (A) the C1/C1inh complex (classical pathway); (B) the C3b,BbP complex (alternative pathway); and (C) the SC5b–9 complex (terminal pathway). P, properdin; C1inh, C1 inhibitor; S, S protein.

### 12.2.5.3 Activation complex of the terminal pathway

The fluid-phase activation complex of the terminal pathway is the SC5b–9 complex. This complex has been detected using antibodies against C5 and C9; however, the high concentrations of the component proteins make it necessary to separate the complex by salt precipitation prior to assay. Sample processing can be eliminated by the use of antineoantigenic antibodies. The SC5b–9 complex expresses several antigenic determinants which are not present on any of the native proteins. Most of these new determinants are derived from C9 within the complex and are also expressed on polymerized C9 and on the membrane attack complex (MAC). A few neoantigenic determinants have been discovered on other components of the complex. Antibodies against these neoantigens have been produced and used as capture antibodies in ELISA assays. Antibody on the plate specifically binds the SC5b–9 complex from the sample, and this can be detected subsequently using an antibody to one of the native components of the complex (Fig. 12.3). All the neoantigenic anti-SC5b–9 antibodies thus far described also recognize the MAC. In some diseases, detectable amounts of the MAC are released into the fluid phase. MAC can be distinguished from SC5b–9 after binding to capture antibody by using anti-S protein as a second antibody, thus detecting only the latter complex. The activation complexes, their uses and advantages are summarized in Table 12.3.

Table 12.3 Activation complexes of complement.

| Complex | Assay method | Comments |
| --- | --- | --- |
| C1/C1inh | ELISA; anti-C1s on plate, anti-C1inh label | Good index of ongoing CP activation, stable *in vitro*, simple assay (no sample preparation) |
| C3b,BpP | ELISA; anti-P on plate, anti-C3 label | Good index of AP activation, stable *in vitro*, simple assay (no sample preparation) |
| SC5b-9 | ELISA; antineoantigenic antibody on plate, antibody against native component as label | Sensitive and specific index of complement activation, demonstrates complete activation of system, very stable complex *in vitro*, simple assay if specific antibodies are available |

CP, Classical pathway; AP, alternative pathway; ELISA, enzyme-linked immunosorbent assay; P, properdin.

### 12.2.6 Complement activation in tissues

Complement activation releases fragments and activation products into the fluid phase, and also causes their deposition in tissues. Localization and/or quantitation of tissue bound complement is a useful adjunct to measurements in biological fluids in those situations where biopsy material is available. The demonstration of complement deposition in tissues at autopsy may also help to establish the relevance of complement to a particular disease process. Deposition of C3 fragments in renal tissue during glomerulonephritis was first noted over 30 years. More recently, highly specific antibodies against native components and against neoantigenic determinants of the activation products have been applied to the study of complement in tissues. Localization of the MAC has proven particularly useful as an index of complement activation. Numerous examples of MAC deposition in renal and other tissues are discussed in earlier chapters. Most studies of complement deposition in tissues have utilized frozen sections in order to maximize detection. The degree of preservation of antigens in fixed and embedded tissue is much lower, and many antibodies consequently work only on unfixed, frozen sections. Despite these technical problems, localization of complement components and fragments in tissue by light or electron microscopy is increasingly performed and used in diagnosis.

## 12.2.7 Which assays and when?

Although the number of complement assays available has increased markedly in recent years, the outcome is simplification rather than complication. It is now relatively easy to state under what circumstance a particular assay or type of assay is likely to be of clinical relevance. Some guidelines to identify the appropriate investigations for a particular clinical problem are listed below. Obviously, a degree of generalization is necessary and the guidelines may not be applicable to every clinical situation.

(1) Measurement of complement lytic activity is a useful screen of the integrity of the system, particularly where a deficiency is suspected.

(2) Functional and immunochemical measurements of individual components are required to confirm or pinpoint a suspected deficiency but are otherwise of little clinical use.

(3) Direct measurement of activation products — either fragments or complexes — is the only way to demonstrate ongoing complement activation.

(4) By measuring appropriate activation products the relative contributions of the two activation pathways and the terminal pathway to the disease process can be determined.

(5) In most situations measurement of activation complexes offers advantages because of their relatively long half-lives *in vivo*, their stability on storage *in vitro*, and the specificity and sensitivity of the assay methods available.

## 12.3 PHARMACOLOGICAL CONTROL OF COMPLEMENT ACTIVATION

The development of nontoxic compounds which specifically modulate the activity of the complement system *in vivo* is of obvious therapeutic relevance. The techniques used to achieve decomplementation in animal models are not suitable for clinical application. Cobra venom factor (CVF) efficiently depletes complement in experimental animals and has been shown to influence greatly the clinical course of several experimental diseases (e.g. experimental myasthenia gravis; see Section 8.2.1). However, CVF is not suitable for clinical use. It activates complement acutely, generating large amounts of active complement fragments, decomplementation is of short duration, and antibodies to CVF are produced, rendering the recipient refractory to repeated treatment.

The quest for compounds capable of specifically inhibiting complement has generated an enormous amount of information on the effects of substances on complement *in vitro* but relatively little data on inhibition *in vivo*. Many compounds have been shown to inhibit the classical and/or the alternative activation pathways *in vitro* (Table 12.4), but the great majority of these substances are

Table 12.4 Pharmacological inhibitors of complement activation.

| Group | Agents | Inhibitory actions* |
|---|---|---|
| *Peptides* | Nonspecific protease inhibitors | Inhibit active site of many proteases, including C enzymes; toxic |
| | Analogues of C1 binding site on IgG | Block binding of C1, thus inhibit CP |
| | Analogues of scission site in C3 | Competitively inhibit activation of C3 by C3 convertases |
| | Analogues of scission site in Factor B | Competitively inhibit activation of Factor B by Factor D |
| *Polyanions* | Carageenan<br>Polyethene sulphate | Inhibit CP and AP activation by interfering at multiple stages |
| | Dextran sulphate<br>Heparin<br>Suramin<br>Polylysine | Inhibit predominantly the CP at multiple stages |
| *Polynucleotides* | Polyinosinic acid<br>Polyguanylic acid | Inhibit CP activation by interfering with C1 attachment |
| *Anti-inflammatory agents* | Steroids | Inhibit AP activation by interfering with assembly of C3 convertase |
| | Nonsteroidal | Inhibit CP by interfering with assembly and enhancing decay of C5 convertase |
| | Gold salts | Inhibit AP by interfering with assembly of C3/C4 convertase |
| *Natural organic compounds* | K-76 COOH | Inhibits CP and AP at multiple stages |

CP, Classical pathway; AP, alternative pathway.
* Most of the actions noted have only been demonstrated *in vitro*.

unsuitable for clinical use because of their toxicity or the impossibility of achieving effective plasma concentrations. The following sections describe some of the groups of compounds and strategies which are of potential therapeutic interest.

### 12.3.1 Peptide inhibitors

Several small peptides have been shown to inhibit complement activity *in vitro*. The tripeptide leupeptin caused marked inhibition of C1s and of several noncomplement serine proteases, and was shown to inhibit cutaneous anaphylactic reactions when instilled locally. More specific inhibitors of complement activation have recently been designed by synthesizing peptides which mimic the sequence around the sites at which components are cleaved during activation. Peptides derived from the sequences of C3 around the site of cleavage by C2, and the sequence of Factor B around the site of cleavage by Factor D have been shown to be potent competitive inhibitors of activation *in vitro*. These peptides should be nontoxic and nonimmunogenic but have not as yet been tested *in vivo*.

### 12.3.2 Inhibition by polyanions

A variety of charged molecules have been shown to inhibit complement activation *in vitro* (Table 12.4). Most of these compounds interfere with activation of C1. Intravenous administration of the sulphated polysaccharide carageenan markedly reduces complement activity in animals, and the antilepromatous drug suramin inhibits complement-mediated tissue injury in rabbits. The *in vivo* effects of the other compounds in this group have not been investigated. The anticomplementary effect of heparin has recently been shown to be influenced by its molecular weight, low-molecular-weight heparin fractions having strong anticomplement but poor anticoagulant activity. Polyanions modified to maximize complement inhibition may therefore prove useful in therapy.

### 12.3.3 Steroids and other anti-inflammatory agents

In patients with ongoing complement activation, pharmacological doses of corticosteroids cause an immediate reduction in the levels of activation products in plasma. *In vitro*, these drugs inhibit the formation of the C3/C5 convertases of both activation pathways. Several nonsteroidal anti-inflammatory drugs, including flufenamic acid and mefenamic acid, inhibit C4 cleavage by C1 *in vitro* and inhibit complement-mediated tissue damage in experimental animals. Gold salts, used therapeutically in the treatment of severe rheumatoid arthritis, also inhibit complement, by accelerating inactivation of C1 and by interfering with the formation of the alternative-pathway C3 convertase.

### 12.3.4 Naturally occurring organic inhibitors

A monocarboxylic acid derivative purified from the fungus *Stachybotrys complementi*, K-76 COOH, is a potent and relatively nontoxic inhibitor of complement activation. It acts at several stages of both activation pathways but has its main effect upon C5. This compound has proven capable of preventing complement-induced tissue damage in several model systems. Its potential as a therapeutic agent in man has not been investigated. The search for other plant- or microorganism-derived inhibitors continues.

### 12.3.5 Therapeutic control of complement activation

Although some of the compounds described above show promise, it is clear that powerful, specific and nontoxic inhibitors of complement activation suitable for use *in vivo* are as yet not available. Research should proceed along two lines: the continued quest for new compounds which inhibit complement *in vitro*; and the examination of drugs in current clinical use for potential complement inhibitory activity.

As emphasized elsewhere in this book, the complement system is a double-edged sword, activation having a protective role in appropriate situations but pathological consequences when inappropriate. Therapeutic inhibition of the complement system will therefore influence the immune status of the patient. In order to achieve clinical benefit it will be necessary to balance these opposing requirements, perhaps by aiming to dampen-down rather than wipe out complement activation. Alternatively, it may be possible to 'target' inhibitory molecules to sites of inflammation, leaving the complement system intact elsewhere (Fig. 12.4). A future strategy could be to use analogues of the naturally occurring inhibitory proteins, perhaps combined with targetting, to decrease activation

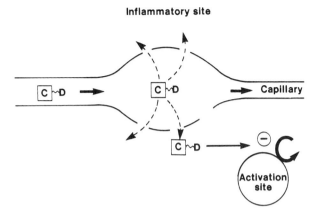

*Figure 12.4* Delivery of complement inhibitor to site of activation.
The figure illustrates one possible strategy for targetting labile or toxic anticomplementary drugs to sites of complement activation. The carrier molecule (C) retains the drug (D) in the circulation until the complex reaches a site of inflammation. Increased capillary permeability at the inflammatory site allows efflux of the complex into the tissues where the drug, either attached to or after release from the carrier, acts to inhibit complement activation and dampen down inflammation.

specifically at inflammatory sites.

We are still some way from being able to modulate the complement system in human disease but it is to be expected that with the increasing interest of the pharmacological industry in complement, suitable agents will soon emerge.

## 12.4 FURTHER READING

*Complement measurement*
Thomson, R. A. (1981). Assessment of clinical hypocomplementaemia. In: *Techniques in Clinical Immunology*. Blackwell Scientific, Oxford. pp. 95–105.
Cooper, N. R., Nemerow, G. R. and Mayes, J. T. (1983). Methods to detect and quantitate complement activation. *Springer Semin. Immunopathol.* **6**, 195–212.
Whaley, K. (1985). Measurement of complement. In: Whaley, K. (ed.), *Methods in Complement for Clinical Immunologists*. Churchill-Livingstone, Edinburgh, pp. 77–139.
Laurell, A.-B. (1988). Complement determinations in clinical diagnosis. In: Rother, K. and Till, G. O. (eds), *The Complement System*. Springer, Berlin, pp. 272–287.
Rauterberg, E. W. (1988). Demonstration of complement deposits in tissue.

In: Rother, K. and Till, G. O. (eds), *The Complement System*. Springer, Berlin, pp. 287–326.

Whaley, K. (1989). Measurement of complement activation in clinical practice. *Complement Inflamm.* **6**, 96–103.

*Therapy*

Asghar, S. S. (1984). Pharmacological manipulation of the complement system. *Pharmacol. Rev.* **36**, 223–244.

Inoue, K. (1988). *In vivo* manipulation of the complement system. In: Rother, K. and Till, G. O. (eds), *The Complement System*. Springer, Berlin, pp. 520–524.

# Index

Activation
 assays of, 194
Activation pathways
 classical,
  historical, 4–5
  components, 9, 12
 alternative,
  historical, 4–6
  components, 9, 18
Acute allergic arthritis
 model for RA, 132
Adult respiratory distress syndrome
  (ARDS)
 complement activation in, 173
 complement assay and, 174
 definition, 173
$AH_{50}$, 194
Alexin, 3
Allotypes (see individual
 components), 57–62
Alternative pathway
 amplification, 20
 assay for activation 195, 196, 200
 components, 18
 control in, 31
 formation of initial convertase, 18
 formation of membrane
  convertase, 19
 haemolysis in, 194
 historical, 4–5
Alzheimer's disease, 151
Amplification
 in alternative pathway, 20

in classical pathway, 12
Anabolic steroids
 treatment of HAE, 88
Anaphylatoxins
 assay, 197
 control of, 37
 in ARDS, 173
 in CPB, 172
 in haemodialysis, 170
 receptors for, 38
 relative potencies, 37
Anaphylaxis
 definition, 37
 historical, 7
Angioedema
 acquired, 88
 hereditary, 87
 other, 163
Antibody response, 52
Anti-GBM nephritis, 114
Anti-TBM nephritis, 117
Arachidonic acid metabolites
 C5a and production of, 41
 MAC and production of, 42
 role in inflammation, 118, 135
Atheroma, 179
Autoimmune haemolytic anaemia
 (see haemolytic anaemia)

B (see Factor B)
Ba
 chemotactic activity, 40
 formation, 19

measurement of, 198
Bacteria
  structure and complement activation, 103
Bactericidal activity, 2, 104
Bayer's adhesion zones, 106
B cells
  and complement in antibody response, 52
  proliferation and angioedema, 88
Behcet's disease, 137
Berger's disease (IgA nephropathy), 120
Bioincompatibility, 169
Biosyntheseis of complement components, 75–80
Bordet, Jules, 2
Bradykinin
  role in HAE, 88
Buchner, Hans, 2
Bullous pemphigoid, 158
Bystander lysis, 22

C1
  activation, 13
  chromosomal assignment, 77
  deficiency, 81
  structure, 12
C1r/C1s
  chromosomal assignment, 77
  deficiencies, 81
  genetic linkage, 64
  homology, 64
C1 inhibitor
  acquired deficiency, 88
  and angioedema, 88
  chromosomal assignment, 77
  congenital deficiency, 87
  structure and function, 29
C2
  chromosomal assignment, 77
  deficiency, 82
  kinin in HAE, 88
  polymorphisms in, 60
  structure and activation, 1
C3
  chromosomal assignment, 77
  deficiency, 84
  fragments, 17, 46
  homologies with C4 and C5, 66
  polymorphisms in, 61
  structure and activation, 15
C3a
  anaphylactic activity, 37
  chemotactic activity, 40
  formation, 15
  measurement, 197
C3b
  receptors for, 46
  role in opsonisation, 44
C3 nephritic factor, 94
C4
  chromosomal assignment, 77
  deficiency, 83
  homologies with C3 and C5, 66
  polymorphisms in, 60
  structure and activation, 14
C4a
  anaphylactic activity, 37
  formation, 14
C4A
  binding characteristics, 60
  blood group associations, 60
  deficiency, 83, 126
C4 allotypes, 60
C4b
  formation, 14
  receptors for, 46
  role in opsonisation, 45
C4B
  binding characteristics, 60
  blood group associations, 60
  deficiency, 83
C4 binding protein (C4bp)
  chromosomal assignment, 77
  presence in RCA cluster, 67
  structure and function, 30
C5
  acid/freeze-thaw activation, 16
  chromosomal assignment, 77
  deficiency, 85
  homologies with C3 and C4, 66
  structure and activation, 16, 20
C5a
  anaphylactic activity, 37
  chemotactic activity, 40
  formation, 16, 20
  measurement of, 197
  neutrophil activation by, 41
  receptors for, 38
C5b6, 6
C5b-9 (see membrane attack complex)
C6
  deficiency, 85
  polymorphisms in, 62
  structure and function, 21

Index 211

C7
  deficiency, 85
  polymorphisms in, 62
  structure and function, 21
C8
  deficiency, 85
  polymorphisms in, 62
  structure and function, 22
C9
  deficiency, 85
  in Behcet's disease, 137
  homology with perforin, 70
  structure and function, 22
Carboxypeptidase N (anaphylatoxin inactivator), 37, 40
Cardiopulmonary bypass (CPB), 172
Cell-mediated lysis, 28
$CH_{50}$, 194
Chemotaxis
  complement-derived factors, 40
  definition, 38
Chido and Rogers blood groups, 60
Class III MHC, 65
Classical pathway
  assays for activation, 195, 196, 199
  C1 activation in, 12
  components, 9
  control in, 28
  haemolysis in, 194
  historical, 4
Clearance
  of immune complexes, 49–51
  of microorganisms, 100, 104
Cobra venom factor (CVF)
  mechanism of action, 52, 103
  use in animal models, 113, 117, 132, 142, 147, 162
Coeliac disease, 185
Collagen-induced arthritis Type II, 131–132
Complement activation
  assays for, 194
  by antibody, 12
  by foreign surfaces, 18
  complexes, 199
  IgG subclasses and, 13
Complement assay, 194–201
Complement cleavage products
  assay, 196
  anaphylatoxins, 37
  chemotaxins, 38
  opsonins, 43
Complement deficiencies (see individual components), 80–95
Complement receptors
  and SLE, 127
  C3a/C5a, 38
  C3b and fragments, 46
Coombs test, 186
CR1
  deficiency, 91
  and SLE, 127
  structure and distribution, 46
CR2, 46
CR3
  deficiency, 91
  structure and distribution, 47
CR4 (p150, 95), 47
Crohn's disease, 184
Cryoglobulinaemia, 139
Cysteine-rich domains, 71–75
Cytolysin (see also perforin), 72

D (see Factor D)
Decay accelerating factor (DAF)
  presence in RCA cluster, 66
  role in PNH, 92
  structure and function, 30
Demyelination
  by complement in vitro, 145
  in multiple sclerosis, 144
Dengue haemorrhagic fever, 103
Dermatitis herpetiformis, 161
Dermatomyositis, 151
Diabetes mellitus, 184
Discoid lupus erythematosus (DLE), 165
Disseminated intravascular coagulation (DIC), 175
Doughnut hypothesis, 7
Drugs
  activation of complement by, 176
  and haemolysis, 188
  and SLE, 128
  as inhibitors of complement, 203

E-aminocaproic acid (EACA), 88
Ehrlich, Paul, 3
Eicosanoids
  C5a and production of, 41
  MAC and production of, 42
  role in inflammation, 118, 135
Endpiece, 4
Epstein-Barr virus (EBV)
  complement neutralization, 100
  interaction with CR2, 47

Erythrocyte
  clearance, 186
  immune complex transport, 50
  lysis by MAC, 26
Experimental allergic
  encephalomyelitis (EAE), 146
Experimental autoimmune
  myasthenia gravis (EAMG),
  142

Factor A, 5
Factor B
  historical, 5
  polymorphisms in, 62
  structure and activation, 19
Factor D, 19
Factor H
  deficiency, 90
  structure and function, 32
Factor I
  deficiency, 89
  structure and function, 30
Factor P (see properdin)
Fibronectin, 43
Follicular dendritic cells, 54
Freeze-thaw activation, 16
Fungal infections and complement, 108

Genes, complement component
  chromosomal assignment, 76
  localization in MHC, 65
  localization in RCA cluster, 66
  mapping of, 76
Genetic deficiencies (see individual
  components), 80–96
Genetic polymorphisms, 57–62
Glomerulonephritis
  and complement deficiency, 81
  animal models, 113–118
  human disease, 118–122
Goodpasture's syndrome, 114
gp45-70 (see MCP)
Gram negative bacteria
  and complement activation, 104
  structure of cell wall, 105
Gram positive bacteria, 105
Granulocyte (see neutrophil)
Graves' disease, 182
Guillain–Barré syndrome, 150

H (see Factor H)
Haemodialysis
  activator membranes, 171
  and complement activation, 170
Haemolytic anaemia
  complement in, 186
  definition, 185
  drug-induced, 188
Haemolytic assays, 194
Hashimoto's thyroiditis, 182
Heparin, 205
Hereditary angioedema (HAE), 87–89
Hereditary erythroblastic
  multinuclearity with positive
  acidified serum lysis
  (HEMPAS), 93
Herpes gestationis, 161
Herpes simplex virus, 100
Heymann nephritis, 115
Histamine, 38
High density lipoprotein (HDL), 33
Homologies in the complement
  system
  C1r and C1s, 64
  C2 and Factor B, 64
  C3, C4 and C5, 66
  C9 and perforin, 70
  RCA cluster, 66
  Terminal components, 68
Hydralazine, 128
21-hydroxylase, 65
Hypocomplementaemia
  in acute post-streptococcal
  nephritis, 121
  in IgA nephropathy, 120
  in membranoproliferative
  glomerulonephritis, 121
  in parasitic infections, 110
  in Sjogren's syndrome, 136
  in SLE, 123

I (see Factor I)
IgA
  in coeliac disease, 185
  in dermatitis herpetiformis, 161
  in nephritis, 120
IgE, 37
IgG
  subclasses and C1q binding, 13
IgM, 13
Immune adherence, 7
Immune complexes
  and SLE, 123
  binding to erythrocytes, 50
  in renal disease, 112
  solubilization and transport, 47–51

Immune response, complement in, 52–54
Immunological memory, complement and, 53
Infections
 and complement deficiencies, 81–89
Inflammatory bowel disease, 184–185
Internal thiolester
 in C3 and C4, 14–16
Isoelectric focussing, 58
Isoniazid, 128

K-76 COOH, 206
Kinin, 88

Leucocytosis, 41
Leukotriene (see eicosanoid)
LFA-1
 association with CR3, 47
 deficiency, 91
Lipopolysaccharide (LPS), 103
Lung injury
 complement and, 190
 in ARDS, 173
Lupus erythematosus (see systemic lupus erythematosus)
Lymphocyte
 complement and antibody response, 52
 proliferation and angioedema, 88
Lymphoproliferative disorders
 and angioedema, 88
Lysozyme, 106

MAC (see membrane attack complex)
$\alpha_2$-macroglobulin, 66
Macrophage, 50
Major histocompatibility complex (MHC), 65
Malaria, 109
Mapping of complement genes, 76
Mast cells, 37
Membrane attack complex
 active removal of, 26
 and bacterial killing, 105
 and viral killing, 101
 assembly, 21
 comparison with perforin, 28
 evolution, 71
 historical, 6
 in atheroma and infarcts, 179, 181

in bioincompatibility, 172
in dermatological disease, 157, 161, 164
inhibitory proteins, 33
in endocrine diseases, 182–183
in neurological disease, 143, 144, 146–148, 151
in renal diseases, 114–117
in rheumatoid disease, 132, 134, 137
lysis by, 25
structure, 22
Membrane attack pathway
 components, 21
 control in, 33
Membrane cofactor protein (MCP)
 localization in RCA cluster, 66
 structure and function, 30
Membranoproliferative glomerulonephritis (MPGN)
 association with partial lipodystrophy, 121
 nephritic factors and, 93
 Type II, 121,
 Type III, 122
Membranous nephropathy
 animal model, 115
 human disease, 122
Meningitis
 and properdin deficiency, 84
 and terminal component deficiency, 85
Metchnikoff, Eli, 2
Midpiece, 4
MHC (see major histocompatibility complex)
Modular fusion hypothesis, 75
Muir, Robert, 3
Multiple sclerosis (MS)
 definition, 144
 in vitro/animal models, 146
 role of complement, 148
Myasthenia gravis (MG)
 animal model, 142
 definition, 141
 human disease, 143
 MAC in, 144
Myocardial infarction (MI), 181
Myositis (see polymyositis)

Neisserial infections
 properdin deficiency and, 84
 terminal component deficiency and, 85

## 214  Index

Neoantigens, 196
Nephritic factors, 93
Neutrophils
  activation by C5a, 41
  activation by the MAC, 42
  in ARDS, 174
  in pemphigoid, 161
Nomenclature, 4
Nucleocapsid, 98
Null alleles of C4, 59

One hit hypothesis, 26
Opsonization
  C3 derived opsonins, 44
  C4 derived opsonins, 45
  definition, 43
  historical, 8
  in bacterial killing, 104
  in virus kiling, 101
  non-complement, 43
Oxygen radicals (see reactive oxygen metabolites)

P (see properdin)
Parasitic infections
  complement killing in, 108
  immune complexes and, 110
Paroxysmal nocturnal haemoglobinuria (PNH)
  association with DAF deficiency, 92
  defect in MAC control, 92
  description, 91, 185
Partial lipodystrophy
  association with nephritic factor, 94, 166
  membranoproliferative glomerulonephritis and, 121
Pemphigoid, 158
Pemphigus vulgaris, 157
Peptide inhibitors, 205
Perforin
  homology with C9, 70
  role in cell mediated killing, 28
Pfeiffer, Richard, 3
Phagocytosis, 43
Pillemer, Louis, 5
Platelet
  abnormalities in PNH, 93
  removal by complement, 189
Poly-C9, 24
Polymyositis, 151
Polymorphisms of complement components, 57–62

Polytrauma and complement activation, 175–176
Porphyria, 162
Post-streptococcal nephritis
  animal model, 114
  human disease, 121
Pre-eclampsia, 190
Properdin
  deficiency, 84
  historical, 5
  structure and function, 32
  Type I domains in, 75
Prostaglandins (see eicosanoids)
Pseudoallergic reactions, 177
Psoriasis
  arthritis, 137
  skin lesions, 167
Pulmonary disease, 190

Radiographic contrast media, 177
Reactive lysis, 6
Reactive oxygen metabolites
  anaphylatoxins and, 41
  in ARDS, 174
  MAC and, 43
Receptors for complement fragments, 46–49
Regulators of complement activation (RCA) cluster, 66
Retroviruses, 100–101
Rheumatoid arthritis
  animal models for, 131–132
  complement profile in, 135
  definition, 133
  juvenile, 136
Rheumatoid factor, 133
Rocket electrophoresis
  complement assay, 195
  double-decker, 198

SC5b-9 complex (see also terminal complement complex)
  control and, 33
  measurement, 200
Schistosomes, 108
Sensitizer, 3
Sequence homology (see homology)
Serum resistance/sensitivity, 105
Serum sickness glomerulonephritis, 113
Short consensus repeat (SCR), 71
Solubilization of immune complexes, 49
SP-40,40, 33

S protein, 33
Subacute sclerosing
  encephalomyelitis (SSPE), 150
Systemic lupus erythematosus (SLE)
  complement deficiency and, 81, 125
  complement profile in, 123
  complement receptors and, 127
  drugs and, 128
  multi-organ involvement, 123–129

T cell perforins, 28
Terminal complement complex (TCC)
  in ARDS, 174
  in multiple sclerosis, 148
  in rheumatoid arthritis, 133
  in SLE, 123
  in thyroid disease, 183
  measurement of, 200
Thiolester bond, 14, 16
Thrombocytopenia, 189
Transfusion reactions, 187

Trypanosoma, 109
Tubulointerstitial nephritis
  animal model, 115
  human disease, 119

Ulcerative colitis, 184
Urticaria, 163

Vascular permeability, 38
Vasculitis
  complement and, 138
  cutaneous, 163
Vasodilatation, 36
Viruses
  complement activation, 99
  neutralization by complement, 100
  structure and replication, 97
  virus-infected cells, 102

Zymosan
  alternative pathway activation by, 5
  complement receptors and, 47